Otolaryngology

Editor

LAURA A. KIRK

PHYSICIAN ASSISTANT CLINICS

www.physicianassistant.theclinics.com

Consulting Editor
JAMES A. VAN RHEE

April 2018 • Volume 3 • Number 2

ELSEVIER

1600 John F. Kennedy Boulevard • Suite 1800 • Philadelphia, Pennsylvania, 19103-2899

http://www.theclinics.com

PHYSICIAN ASSISTANT CLINICS Volume 3, Number 2
April 2018 ISSN 2405-7991, ISBN-13: 978-0-323-58320-6

Editor: Jessica McCool
Developmental Editor: Casey Potter

Physician Assistant Clinics (ISSN: 2405–7991) is published quarterly by Elsevier Inc., 360 Park Avenue South, New York, NY 10010-1710. Months of issue are January, April, July, and October. Periodicals postage paid at New York, NY and additional mailing offices. Subscription prices are $150.00 per year (US individuals), $205.00 (US institutions), $100.00 (US students), $150.00 (Canadian individuals), $257.00 (Canadian institutions), $100.00 (Canadian students), $150.00 (international individuals), $257.00 (international institutions), and $100.00 (international students). Foreign air speed delivery is included in all *Clinics* subscription prices. All prices are subject to change without notice. POSTMASTER: Send address changes to *Physician Assistant Clinics*, Elsevier Periodicals Customer Service, 11830 Westline Industrial Drive, St. Louis, MO 63146. Customer Service Health Sciences Division, Subscription Customer Service, 3251 Riverport Lane, Maryland Heights, MO 63043. **Customer Service: 1-800-654-2452 (U.S. and Canada); 314-447-8871 (outside U.S. and Canada). Fax: 314-447-8029. E-mail: journalscustomerservice-usa@elsevier.com (for print support); journalsonlinesupport-usa@elsevier.com (for online support).**

Reprints. For copies of 100 or more, of articles in this publication, please contact the Commercial Reprints Department, Elsevier Inc., 360 Park Avenue South, New York, NY 10010-1710. Tel. 212-633-3874; Fax: 212-633-3820; E-mail: reprints@elsevier.com.

Physician Assistant Clinics is covered in *EMBASE/Excerpta Medica* and *ESCI*.

PROGRAM OBJECTIVE

The goal of the *Physician Assistant Clinics* is to keep practicing physician assistants up to date with current clinical practice by providing timely articles reviewing the state of the art in patient care.

TARGET AUDIENCE

Physician Assistants and other healthcare professionals.

LEARNING OBJECTIVES

Upon completion of this activity, participants will be able to:

1. Review pediatric otitis media and sudden sensorineural loss in primary care.
2. Discuss vestibular migraines, sinusitis versus migraine, and benign paryoxysmal positional vertigo.
3. Recognize the evaluation and management of adult neck masses and pediatric neck masses.

ACCREDITATION

The Elsevier Office of Continuing Medical Education (EOCME) is accredited by the Accreditation Council for Continuing Medical Education (ACCME) to provide continuing medical education for physicians.

The EOCME designates this enduring material for a maximum of 15 *AMA PRA Category 1 Credit*(s)™. Physicians should claim only the credit commensurate with the extent of their participation in the activity.

All other health care professionals requesting continuing education credit for this enduring material will be issued a certificate of participation.

DISCLOSURE OF CONFLICTS OF INTEREST

The EOCME assesses conflict of interest with its instructors, faculty, planners, and other individuals who are in a position to control the content of CME activities. All relevant conflicts of interest that are identified are thoroughly vetted by EOCME for fair balance, scientific objectivity, and patient care recommendations. EOCME is committed to providing its learners with CME activities that promote improvements or quality in healthcare and not a specific proprietary business or a commercial interest.

The planning committee, staff, authors and editors listed below have identified no financial relationships or relationships to products or devices they or their spouse/life partner have with commercial interest related to the content of this CME activity:

Holly J. Baker, MHS, PA-C; Jeff E. Brockett, EdD, CCC-A; Joseph Daniel; Denise L. Jackson, PA-C, MA, CCC-SLP; William J. Jensen, PA-C, MMS; Jennifer Johnson, MPAS, PA-C; Alison Kemp; Laura A. Kirk, MSPAS, PA-C; Roseanne Krauter, FNP-BC; Kimberly J.T. Lakhan, DHSc, MPAS, PA-C; Leah Logan, MBA; Jessica McCool; Alan K. Mirly, MBA, PA-C; Casey Potter; Jeffrey M. Robin, MSHS, PA-C; Robert T. Sataloff, MD, DMA, FACS; Trina M. Sheedy, MMS, PA-C; Linda J. Smith, MPAS, PA-C; James A. Van Rhee, MS, PA-C.

The planning committee, staff, authors and editors listed below have identified financial relationships or relationships to products or devices they or their spouse/life partner have with commercial interest related to the content of this CME activity:

N/A

UNAPPROVED/OFF-LABEL USE DISCLOSURE

The EOCME requires CME faculty to disclose to the participants:

1. When products or procedures being discussed are off-label, unlabelled, experimental, and/or investigational (not US Food and Drug Administration [FDA] approved); and
2. Any limitations on the information presented, such as data that are preliminary or that represent ongoing research, interim analyses, and/or unsupported opinions. Faculty may discuss information about pharmaceutical agents that is outside of FDA-approved labelling. This information is intended solely for CME and is not intended to promote off-label use of these medications. If you have any questions, contact the medical affairs department of the manufacturer for the most recent prescribing information.

TO ENROLL

The CME program is available to all *Physician Assistant Clinics* subscribers at no additional fee. To subscribe to the *Physician Assistant Clinics*, call customer service at 1-800-654-2452 or sign up online at www.physicianassistant.theclinics.com.

METHOD OF PARTICIPATION

In order to claim credit, participants must complete the following:

1. Complete enrolment as indicated above.
2. Read the activity.
3. Complete the CME Test and Evaluation. Participants must achieve a score of 70% on the test. All CME Tests and Evaluations must be completed online.

CME INQUIRIES/SPECIAL NEEDS

For all CME inquiries or special needs, please contact elsevierCME@elsevier.com.

Contributors

CONSULTING EDITOR

JAMES A. VAN RHEE, MS, PA-C
Associate Professor, Program Director, Yale School of Medicine, Yale Physician Assistant Online Program, New Haven, Connecticut

EDITOR

LAURA A. KIRK, MSPAS, PA-C
Senior Physician Assistant, Supervisor, Department of Otolaryngology–Head and Neck Surgery, UCSF Medical Center, San Francisco, California

AUTHORS

HOLLY J. BAKER, MHS, PA-C
Physician Assistant, ENT and Allergy Specialists, Instructor, Department of Otolaryngology–Head and Neck Surgery, Drexel University College of Medicine, Philadelphia, Pennsylvania

JEFF E. BROCKETT, EdD, CCC-A
Associate Professor of Audiology, Department of Communication Sciences and Disorders, Idaho State University, Pocatello, Idaho

DENISE L. JACKSON, PA-C, MA, CCC-SLP
Physician Assistant, Speech Language Pathologist, Otolaryngology–Head and Neck Surgery, University of Virginia Medical Center, Charlottesville, Virginia

WILLIAM J. JENSEN, PA-C, MMS
Physician Assistant, Pediatric Otolaryngology, Saint Alphonsus Regional Medical Center, Boise, Idaho

JENNIFER JOHNSON, MPAS, PA-C
Director of Simulation Education, Principal Faculty, Assistant Professor, Physician Assistant Program, Rocky Mountain University of Health Professions, Provo, Utah

LAURA A. KIRK, MSPAS, PA-C
Senior Physician Assistant, Supervisor, Department of Otolaryngology–Head and Neck Surgery, UCSF Medical Center, San Francisco, California

ROSEANNE KRAUTER, FNP-BC
Nurse Practitioner III, Department of Otolaryngology–Head and Neck Surgery, UCSF Medical Center, Assistant Clinical Professor, Department of Family Health Care Nursing, UCSF School of Nursing, San Francisco, California

KIMBERLY J.T. LAKHAN, DHSc, MPAS, PA-C
Assistant Professor, Department of Physician Assistant Studies, The College of
St. Scholastica, Physician Assistant, Department of Otolaryngology, Essentia
Health-Duluth Clinic, Duluth, Minnesota

ALAN K. MIRLY, MBA, PA-C
Pocatello Ear, Nose & Throat, Assistant Professor, Department of Physician Assistant
Studies, Idaho State University, Pocatello, Idaho

JEFFREY M. ROBIN, MSHS, PA-C
Physician Assistant-Certified, Head and Neck/Endocrine Surgery, Swedish Cancer
Institute, Seattle, Washington

ROBERT T. SATALOFF, MD, DMA, FACS
Professor and Chairman, Department of Otolaryngology–Head and Neck Surgery, Senior
Associate Dean for Clinical Academic Specialties, Drexel University College of Medicine,
Philadelphia, Pennsylvania

TRINA M. SHEEDY, MMS, PA-C
Physician Assistant, Head and Neck Surgical Oncology, Department of
Otolaryngology–Head and Neck Surgery, University of California San Francisco,
San Francisco, California

LINDA J. SMITH, MPAS, PA-C
Department of Head and Neck Surgery, Kaiser Permanente, San Diego, California

Contents

Foreword: New Year Resolutions   xiii

James A. Van Rhee

Preface: Otolaryngology: A Selection of Diverse and Relevant Topics for Primary Care   xv

Laura A. Kirk

Benign Paroxysmal Positional Vertigo: State-of-the-"Art" Diagnosis and Treatment   149

Linda J. Smith

Dizziness accounts for approximately 5% of annual primary care clinic visits, with approximately 20% of those visits due to benign paroxysmal positional vertigo (BPPV). The lifetime prevalence of BPPV is 2.4%, most commonly occurring in the fifth to seventh decades. Delay in diagnosis and treatment can last months, often with unnecessary medications or diagnostic testing, which has associated cost and quality-of-life implications. When properly diagnosed with directed history and examination, including Dix-Hallpike or supine roll maneuver testing, appropriate treatment with repositioning maneuvers or exercises can be given, often facilitating swift resolution of symptoms.

Vestibular Migraine: Diagnostic Criteria and Treatment Options   163

Roseanne Krauter

Vestibular migraine is described in medical texts as far back as the second century. Despite the enduring awareness of this disorder, little remains known about the pathophysiology and optimal treatment for vestibular migraine. It is known that vestibular migraine is common with a 1.0% to 3.2% lifetime prevalence. Preliminary studies have been completed to describe the efficacy of commonly used migraine medication for vestibular migraine. There is a need for well-designed randomized controls trials and a standardized outcomes measure tool to provide direction for providers in the treatment of vestibular migraine.

"Sinus" Headaches: Sinusitis Versus Migraine   181

Kimberly J.T. Lakhan

Sinus symptoms are one of the nation's top health care complaints and top diagnoses for antibiotic usage. Yet viruses, not bacteria, are by far the most common cause of acute rhinosinusitis, accounting for most acute sinus infections. There is significant overlap between viral and acute bacterial rhinosinusitis, chronic rhinosinusitis, and migraine. Thus, antibiotics should not be used unless criteria for acute bacterial rhinosinusitis are met. Migraine should be considered in those patients with chronic and recurrent "sinus" headache who complain of recurrent sinus pain/pressure and nasal congestion, especially when other findings are lacking or when symptoms do not improve with traditional sinus modalities.

Pediatric Sleep-Disordered Breathing   193

William J. Jensen

> Inquiries are often made by caregivers in pediatric and primary care settings regarding the need for tonsillectomy. Sleep-disordered breathing (SDB) is the predominant indication for tonsillectomy in children. SDB and its sequelae are well documented as having a negative impact on several domains of a child's life and should be considered within the differential diagnosis for several common pediatric conditions. A diagnosis of SDB is generally made through a thorough history and physical examination. There is evidence for the benefit of adenotonsillectomy for children with SDB and for recurrent throat infections in the short term, but studies with longer-term outcomes are lacking.

Pediatric Otitis Media: An Update   207

Laura A. Kirk

> Pediatric otitis media affects most children at some point. Although there are clear and updated clinical practice guidelines available regarding the diagnosis and management of pediatric otitis media, findings show that the practice patterns of many clinicians who care for pediatric patients do not align with these evidence-based recommendations. This article explains the pathophysiology and impact of otitis media, provides diagnostic pearls, differentiates between acute otitis media and otitis media with effusion, and presents recommendations for optimal diagnosis and treatment according to the various relevant clinical practice guidelines. Directions of current and future research regarding pediatric otitis media are also presented.

Cochlear Implants in the Elderly: Recognizing a Frequently Missed Demographic of Surgical Candidates for Hearing Restoration   223

Holly J. Baker and Robert T. Sataloff

> Of the population over 70 years, 50% to 60% experience hearing impairment. Presbycusis is the most common etiology. Traditional hearing aids may not provide sufficient amplification. Sensorineural hearing loss usually cannot be reversed. Health care providers must recognize treatment modalities that might improve quality of life, including cochlear implants. Although substantial benefits and limited risks are associated with cochlear implantation, there remain a significant number of unrecognized potential candidates. Medical professionals have a shared responsibility to inform patients of all options for hearing rehabilitation, which requires understanding criteria for cochlear implants candidacy and understanding the potential benefits of cochlear implants.

Sudden Sensorineural Loss in Primary Care: An Often-Missed Diagnosis   235

Alan K. Mirly and Jeff E. Brockett

> Idiopathic sudden sensorineural hearing loss (ISSNHL) is a common problem with a reported incidence of between 5 and 27 per 100,000 individuals per year, but some estimates are as high as 160 per 100,000. This discrepancy, and likely underreporting, is due to patients with rapid improvement not presenting for evaluation and treatment. For example, aural fullness is

a common presenting symptom, which is easy to attribute to other conditions. It is important to consider an ISSNHL in any patient presenting with aural fullness because early diagnosis and treatment improves the prognosis for hearing recovery.

Evaluation and Management of Pediatric Neck Masses: An Otolaryngology Perspective   245

Denise L. Jackson

Most pediatric neck masses encountered in primary care are benign, reactive lymph nodes that originate from common pediatric viral processes. In a pediatric otolaryngology practice, more unusual pathologies are encountered, such as embryologic anomalies, vascular lesions, or neoplasms. Lesions that are larger or that have concerning features will ultimately need imaging and excisional biopsy for histopathologic confirmation of the diagnosis. A sound clinician understanding of anatomic neck spaces and common etiologies of pediatric neck masses can greatly reduce nonessential testing, cost, delay in treatment, and parental angst.

Evaluation and Management of Adult Neck Masses   271

Trina M. Sheedy

The epidemiology of neck masses in adults in the primary or acute care setting is relatively unknown. The assumption is that most neck masses are reactive lymphadenopathy secondary to infectious or inflammatory processes. Providers should be suspicious of malignant disease when an adult older than 40 years presents with a neck mass. With the increasing incidence of human papillomavirus–related oropharyngeal carcinoma, the primary care setting could see an influx of adults with a seemingly benign neck mass actually presenting with metastatic cancer. This is an epidemiologic shift within the otolaryngology specialty; thus, frontline providers should understand the change as well.

Ear, Nose, and Throat Manifestations of Sarcoidosis   285

Jennifer Johnson

Sarcoidosis is a multisystem disease that can be difficult to diagnose. Although pulmonary structures are most commonly involved, sarcoidosis often involves structures of the head and neck. Initial misdiagnosis is common, necessitating tissue biopsy and radiologic imaging modalities to arrive at a correct diagnosis. Of head and neck manifestations, the most common subsite is cervical lymph nodes. Other subsites discussed in this article include the larynx, sinonasal region, salivary gland, ear, and pituitary gland. Systemic corticosteroids are the mainstay of treatment for most ear, nose, and throat manifestations.

Primary Hyperparathyroidism   297

Jeffrey M. Robin

Primary hyperparathyroidism is one of the leading causes of hypercalcemia in outpatients. Manifestations of primary hyperparathyroidism include skeletal and renal disease. The automated serum autoanalyzer increased the diagnostic capacity for primary hyperparathyroidism dramatically. Most patients currently diagnosed with primary hyperparathyroidism are asymptomatic. Minimally invasive parathyroidectomy is the preferred surgical treatment. First-time parathyroid surgery has a success rate as high as 98%. Preoperative localization studies, along with a combination of intraoperative laboratory tests, radioguidance, and pathologic evaluation of abnormal parathyroid tissue, are routinely used. More than one-third of patients with asymptomatic primary hyperparathyroidism have progression of disease without surgical intervention.

PHYSICIAN ASSISTANT CLINICS

FORTHCOMING ISSUES

July 2018
Women's Health
Heather P. Adams and Aleece Fosnight,
Editors

October 2018
Geriatrics
Steven D. Johnson, *Editor*

January 2019
Laboratory Medicine
Jane McDaniel, *Editor*

RECENT ISSUES

January 2018
Urology
Todd J. Doran, *Editor*

October 2017
Cardiology
Daniel T. Thibodeau, *Editor*

July 2017
Emergency Medicine
Fred Wu and Michael E. Winters, *Editors*

RELATED INTEREST

Otolaryngologic Clinics of North America
August 2017 (Vol. 50, Issue 4)
Multidisciplinary Approach to Head and Neck Cancer
Maie A. St. John, *Editor*

THE CLINICS ARE AVAILABLE ONLINE!
Access your subscription at:
www.theclinics.com

Foreword
New Year Resolutions

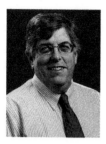

James A. Van Rhee, MS, PA-C
Consulting Editor

As I write this foreword, it is New Year's Day, and I, along with everyone else, am thinking about resolutions. Everyone makes resolutions: lose weight, eat better, or stop smoking. By the second day, we typically have already broken our resolutions. Maybe this year your resolution is to write a journal article. Maybe it is time to write that article about the hypertensive patient you had that was diagnosed with a pheochromocytoma, or maybe you need to write that article for your promotion and reappointment at the university where you work; we all know about the publish or perish philosophy. Well, this journal can help you meet your resolution. If you are interested in writing an article or serving as a guest editor, reach out to me at the e-mail address below under contact information and we can talk about how you can accomplish this New Year resolution.

In this issue, the focus is on otolaryngology. Special thanks to Laura Kirk, from the Department of Otolaryngology–Head and Neck Surgery at the University of California–San Francisco, who serves as the guest editor for this issue. She has put together a number of very interesting articles, covering a wide range of topics, written by excellent authors. This issue really has topics that revisit the basics, like "Pediatric Otitis Media: An Update" by Kirk, "Sinus Headaches" by Lakhan, and an article on Benign Positional Vertigo by Smith, and a number of articles that provide us with the latest information in a variety of some more unusual but very important topics. Cochlear Implants in the Elderly is discussed by Baker and Sataloff; Evaluation and Management of Pediatric Neck Masses is discussed by Jackson, and the ENT Manifestations of Sarcoidosis is discussed by Johnson. You will also enjoy the article on Primary Hyperparathyroidism by Robin, review of Vestibular Migraines by Krauter, Evaluation and Management of Adult Neck Masses by Sheedy, Sudden Sensorineural Loss in Primary Care by Mirly, and Pediatric Sleep-Disordered Breathing by Jensen. As you can see, a wide variety of articles.

Physician Assist Clin 3 (2018) xiii–xiv
https://doi.org/10.1016/j.cpha.2018.01.002
2405-7991/18/© 2018 Published by Elsevier Inc.

physicianassistant.theclinics.com

I hope you enjoy this issue of *Physician Assistant Clinics*. Our next issue will provide you with a review of the latest in women's health.

James A. Van Rhee, MS, PA-C
Yale School of Medicine
Yale Physician Assistant Online Program
100 Church Street South, Suite A230
New Haven, CT 06519, USA

E-mail address:
james.vanrhee@yale.edu

Website:
http://www.paonline.yale.edu

Preface

Otolaryngology: A Selection of Diverse and Relevant Topics for Primary Care

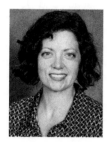

Laura A. Kirk, MSPAS, PA-C
Editor

Otolaryngology, more colloquially known as ENT or Ear, Nose, and Throat, and formally designated as Otolaryngology, Head and Neck Surgery, is a specialty that is often misunderstood by patients and health care colleagues alike. Is otolaryngology a surgical or medical field? The answer is yes, both. Is the domain of an ENT provider primarily ear tubes and tonsillectomies? These are bread-and-butter procedures for otolaryngologists, whose purview is also expansive and fascinating; both common and perhaps surprising conditions that otolaryngology providers treat are well attested to in the diverse offering of articles presented in this issue of *Physician Assistant Clinics*.

Management of common conditions of the ear, nose, throat, and neck that present to primary care providers, urgent care clinics, and emergency departments, such as sinusitis, otitis media, and acute neck lesions, may require referral to an otolaryngologist for expert medical and, when necessary, surgical interventions. Articles in this issue address the nuanced diagnosis and management of each of these conditions, referencing the most up-to-date, evidence-based practice. Dizziness is a particularly perplexing presenting complaint to primary and acute care providers, who will appreciate the thorough and practical discussion of two of the most common causes of dizziness in Linda J. Smith's article, "Benign Paryoxysmal Positional Vertigo: State-of-the-'Art' Diagnosis and Treatment," and Roseanne Krauter's article, "Vestibular Migraine: Diagnostic Criteria and Treatment Options." Providers caring for a pediatric population will find a wealth of guidelines for best practice in William J. Jensen's article, "Pediatric Sleep-Disordered Breathing," and my article. At the other end of the life continuum, internists and gerontologists will find the article exploring advanced options for hearing loss in the elderly, particularly informative (see Holly J. Baker and

Physician Assist Clin 3 (2018) xv–xvi
https://doi.org/10.1016/j.cpha.2018.01.001
2405-7991/18/© 2018 Published by Elsevier Inc.

colleagues' article, "Cochlear Implants in the Elderly: Recognizing a Frequently Missed Demographic of Surgical Candidates for Hearing Restoration"). The distinct and frightening presentation of sudden hearing loss, of utmost importance for all primary care providers to understand, is examined in Alan K. Mirly and Jeff E. Brockett's article, "Sudden Sensorineural Loss in Primary Care: An Often-Missed Diagnosis."

This issue of *Physician Assistant Clinics* illustrates how the regional delineation of Otolaryngology, which addresses most disease processes between the crown of the head to the clavicles, naturally overlaps with many other specialties. Medical and surgical management of infections and masses of the ear, nose, throat, and skin of these areas create collaborative inroads with Infectious Disease and Dermatology fields, as seen in my article, "Pediatric Otitis Media: An Update," Kimberly J.T. Lakhan's article, "'Sinus Headaches': Sinusitis Versus Migraine," Denise L. Jackson's article "Evaluation and Management of Pediatric Neck Masses: An Otolaryngology Perspective," and Trina M. Sheedy's article, "Evaluation and Management of Adult Neck Masses." Otolaryngology clinicians also work closely with neuroradiologists in the diagnosis and surveillance of head and neck masses, as well as differentiating sinus disease from migraine, as seen in Kimberly J.T. Lakhan's article. And complex or refractory headaches are not exclusively the territory of neurologists, as both Kimberly J.T. Lakhan's article and Roseanne Krauter's article beautifully elucidate: most otolaryngologists see ENT manifestations of migraine routinely. Collaboration with rheumatologists is required for patients presenting with sarcoidosis of the sinuses or ears, which are described in Jennifer Johnson's article, "ENT Manifestations of Sarcoidosis," while partnership with endocrinologists is immensely valuable in thyroid and parathyroid diseases, with the latter explored in Jeffrey M. Robin's article, "Primary Hyperparathyroidism."

My coauthors and I believe you will find this varied selection of otolaryngology topics both interesting and relevant to primary care practice, providing plenteous opportunity to enhance and refine treatment of patients of all ages.

Laura A. Kirk, MSPAS, PA-C
Department of Otolaryngology
Head and Neck Surgery
University of California at
San Francisco Medical Center
2380 Sutter Street
San Francisco, CA 94115, USA

E-mail address:
laura.kirk@ucsf.edu

Benign Paroxysmal Positional Vertigo
State-of-the-"Art" Diagnosis and Treatment

Linda J. Smith, MPAS, PA-C

KEYWORDS

- Vertigo • Benign paroxysmal positional vertigo • Vestibular system
- Dix-Hallpike maneuver • Particle repositioning maneuver

KEY POINTS

- Benign paroxysmal positional vertigo (BPPV) is the most common vestibular disorder, but patients may be symptomatic for months without appropriate diagnosis and treatment.
- BPPV most commonly occurs between the fifth and seventh decades of life, increasing the risk of imbalance and subsequent falls for older patients, making proper diagnosis and treatment more important as our population ages.
- Inappropriate diagnostic testing and medications not only contribute to delay of treatment but can also be costly and pose increased risk for patients.
- Once identified with the Dix-Hallpike or supine roll maneuvers, appropriate therapeutic repositioning maneuvers or exercises can facilitate swift resolution of symptoms.

PATHOPHYSIOLOGY

Structures of the inner ear include (**Fig. 1**) the following:

- Bony labyrinth
- Membranous labyrinth
- Vestibule
- Cochlea
- Semicircular canals: posterior, lateral (horizontal), anterior

The bony labyrinth is a shell, which protects the membranous labyrinth, with perilymph fluid filling the space between the two. The vestibule, cochlea, and semicircular canals are structural cavities within the bony labyrinth, containing the organs for hearing (cochlea) and balance (semicircular canals).[1,2]

No disclosures.
Department of Head and Neck Surgery, Kaiser Permanente, 5893 Copley Drive, San Diego, CA 92111, USA
E-mail address: linda.j.smith@kp.org

Physician Assist Clin 3 (2018) 149–162
https://doi.org/10.1016/j.cpha.2017.12.002   physicianassistant.theclinics.com

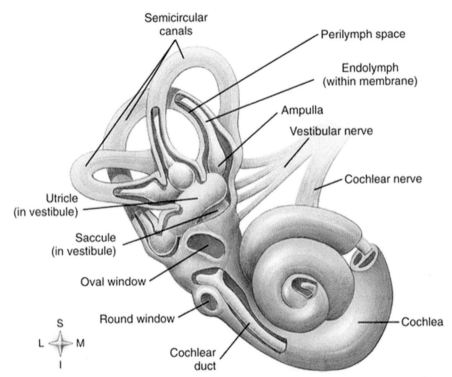

Fig. 1. Inner ear anatomy. (*From* Thibodeau GA, Patton KT: Anatomy and physiology, 6th edition. St Louis: Mosby; 2007. p. 620–657; with permission.)

The vestibular system consists of 3 semicircular canals that are oriented at 90° to each other (the anterior, posterior, and lateral semicircular canals), with their membranous ducts, and the utricle and saccule within the vestibule. The membranous ducts float in perilymph fluid, are continuous with the utricle and saccule, and are filled with endolymph fluid. One end of each canal and duct is enlarged, forming an ampulla. Ampullary crests or cristae and receptor hair cells within the ampulla are embedded in a sugar-protein mass or cupola. As the head turns, movement of endolymph pushes the cristae, thus, bending the hair cells, which fire an impulse that travels through the vestibular portion of cranial nerve VII to the vestibular nuclei of the medulla.

Similar receptor hair cells, or maculae, lie within the utricle and saccule, which lie against the walls of the inner ear between the semicircular ducts and the cochlea. These patches of hair cells are imbedded in a gelatinous layer, topped with calcium salts, called otoliths or otoconia. Movement of the head triggers movement of the endolymph, which pushes the otoliths, thus, bending the hair cells and discharging nerve impulses. The utricle is most sensitive to tilt when the head is upright, and the saccule is most sensitive when the head is horizontal.

The vestibular systems work in pairs detecting head movements: exciting receptors in one ampulla and inhibiting receptors on the opposite side.[1]

PATHOGENESIS OF BENIGN PAROXYSMAL POSITIONAL VERTIGO

- Canalithiasis: Otoconia, which have moved from the utricle and collected near the cupola of the affected semicircular canal, cause the endolymph to abnormally stimulate the vestibular nerve by inertial changes. Nystagmus and vertigo are triggered when the head encounters motion in the plane of the affected semicircular canal.

- Cupulolithiasis: Cristae within the cupula of the affected canal cause abnormal stimulation of the vestibular system.[3]

Benign paroxysmal positional vertigo (BPPV) is usually caused by one of 2 variants:

- Posterior canal BPPV is the most common type, accounting for 85% to 95% of cases, suspected to be due to canalithiasis[4,5]
- Lateral canal BPPV (also known as [aka] horizontal canal BPPV) accounts for 5% to 15% of cases. It is likely due to abnormal debris with the lateral canal but is not as well understood as posterior canal BPPV; it tends to resolve more quickly than posterior canal BPPV and may occur following repositioning maneuvers for the treatment of posterior canal BPPV, known as canal conversion[3,4]
- Rare variations include anterior canal BPPV, multi-canal BPPV, and bilateral multi-canal BPPV and are not addressed.

Fragmentation of the otoconia may occur with aging, contributing to their displacement into the semicircular canals. The peak age for BPPV is about 60 years, with most cases occurring between the fifth and seventh decades of life.[3,4,6] A total of 3.4% of the population older than 60 years has BPPV annually.[4–7] It is seen more commonly in women than men in all age groups, with a reported ratio of 2:1 to 3:1.[4–6] In younger patients, BPPV is the most common type of vertigo seen following a head injury, most likely involving the posterior semicircular canal.[6,8] Posttraumatic BPPV has been found to be more refractory to treatment and may require repeated treatment in up to 67% of cases.[4,6,8]

Case-control studies have found higher relative rates of other comorbidities, which may influence management and treatment outcomes, including the following[4]:

Migraine	34% vs 10% for controls
History of stroke	10% vs 1% for controls
Diabetes	14% vs 5% for controls
Hypertension	52% vs 22% for controls

DIAGNOSIS OF BENIGN PAROXYSMAL POSITIONAL VERTIGO

Once the diagnosis of BPPV has been made, as described later, there is no need for further workup, including radiographic imaging, audiometric testing, or vestibular function testing, such as Vestibular Nystagmography, in the absence of other signs or symptoms inconsistent with BPPV that would warrant further testing.[4]

As in much of medicine, history elicited from patients is often the most important part of the diagnosis. The most common response by patients when asked to describe their symptoms is "I just feel dizzy". The initial challenge to the physician assistant is to try to pin down exactly what patients are experiencing. Vertigo is defined as an "illusory sensation of motion of either the self or the surroundings."[4] Most often this is a sense of spinning or side-to-side movement. In BPPV, patients experience repeated episodes of vertigo triggered by a change in position but may also experience fleeting imbalance with movement without actual spinning, which impacts the gait and increases the fall risk, especially in the older population.[3,4,7] It is important to distinguish vertigo from other types of dizzy causes, such as near-syncope seen in postural hypotension or cardiac issues or gait disturbances, which may be caused by peripheral neuropathy, Parkinson's disease, or stroke.

Questions to ask patients:

- Is there a certain position change that triggers your vertigo?

  BPPV is provoked by a change in head position relative to gravity, unlike Meniere's syndrome, labyrinthitis, or vestibular neuronitis whereby vertigo occurs while still, although may worsen with position change. Simply asking patients if they experience spinning or imbalance after rolling over in bed may help narrow down the diagnosis. If the answer is yes, then question which side is more likely to cause the vertigo. The ear that is down when experiencing the vertigo is more likely the trigger, although occasionally it can occur bilaterally.[3,4] BPPV commonly occurs when patients are tilting the head to look upward (higher shelves) or bending down as in tying shoes. Women may often report vertigo after laying back for hair washing in salons, and men often report vertigo after bending over and tilting to look under a sink or hood of the car.

  Approximately 50% of patients also experience imbalance when walking between the discrete episode of vertigo.[4]

- How long does the spinning last?

  Vertigo with BPPV usually lasts less than 1 minute.[3,4] This distinguishes it from other types of vertigo such as Meniere's syndrome in which the vertigo lasts 30 minutes or longer, or labyrinthitis or vestibular neuronitis where the vertigo may last for several days nonstop. Also, there is often a lag time or latency period from the time of the position change to the onset of vertigo from 5 to 20 seconds, which may be noted by patients: "I moved and thought I was ok, but then the spinning began."[4]

- Do you notice any hearing change, tinnitus, or ear pressure with the vertigo?

  BPPV will not trigger other ear symptoms, such as hearing loss, tinnitus, or otalgia, unlike that which may occur with Meniere's syndrome or labyrinthitis.[4]

PHYSICAL EXAMINATION
Posterior Canal Benign Paroxysmal Positional Vertigo

The Dix-Hallpike maneuver is the gold standard for diagnosing posterior canal BPPV.[4,9] There should be a latency period following completion of the maneuver and onset of subjective vertigo and the objective nystagmus, ranging from 5 to 20 seconds. The subjective vertigo and the nystagmus should start gently, then increase in intensity and gradually decline in intensity as they resolve, in a crescendo-decrescendo fashion, within 60 seconds from the onset of the nystagmus. There is a characteristic mix of torsional and vertical or up-beating movement to the fast component of the nystagmus, with the upper pole of the eye beating toward the dependent ear when the provoking ear is triggered.[3,4,9]

Performing the Dix-Hallpike maneuver (**Fig. 2**)

- Begin with the patient in the upright seated position with the examiner standing at the patient's side. Eyeglasses should be removed. Instruct the patient to keep his or her eyes open, and explain the positional changes that will occur, warning that this may trigger vertigo.
- Rotate the patient's head 45° to the side being tested in order to align the posterior semicircular canal with the midsagittal plane of the body. Move the patient quickly to the supine ear-down position, extending the neck slightly, to about 20° below the horizontal plane of the examining table, with the head continuing to be supported by the examiner. Observe the patient's eyes for latency and the

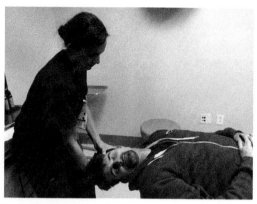

Fig. 2. Performing the Dix-Hallpike maneuver.

duration and direction of the nystagmus, and ask the patient if he or she is experiencing any vertigo (see **Fig. 2**).
- After the subjective vertigo and the nystagmus have resolved, return patient slowly to the upright position and allow any vertigo triggered by the return to resolve before repeating the maneuver to the opposite side.

A negative Dix-Hallpike maneuver does not completely rule out the diagnosis of posterior canal BPPV because studies have reported a positive predictive value of 83% and a negative predictive value of 52%.[4] Factors possibly affecting the diagnostic accuracy of the Dix-Hallpike maneuver include the speed at which the maneuver is performed, the angle of the occipital plane during the maneuver, and even the time of day.[4]

The Dix-Hallpike maneuver should be performed with extra caution or avoided in certain conditions, including the following[4]:

- Significant vascular disease (potential risk of vascular injury or stroke with neck extension in these patients)
- Cervical stenosis or limited cervical range of motion
- Down syndrome
- Low back dysfunction
- Morbid obesity (examiner may require assistance to support the head and position patients for the maneuver)

Lateral (Horizontal) Canal Benign Paroxysmal Positional Vertigo

If the Dix-Hallpike maneuver is negative, and lateral semicircular canal BPPV is suspected, a supine roll test should be performed.[3,4,10] The nystagmus elicited by the test is predominantly horizontal, distinguishing it from the nystagmus seen in the Dix-Hallpike maneuver, which is torsional and up-beating. The vertigo and nystagmus are provoked by turning the head side to side while the patient is supine (**Fig. 3**).

- Begin with the patient supine with the head in the neutral position. Eyeglasses should be removed. Instruct the patient to keep his or her eyes open; explain the positional change that will occur, warning the patient that this may trigger vertigo.

Quickly rotate the patient's head 90° to one side, observing the patient's eyes for nystagmus. After nystagmus subsides, return the patient's head to the face-up supine

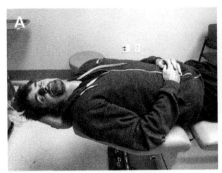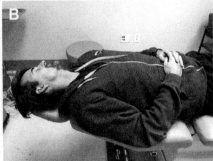

Fig. 3. (*A, B*) Performing supine roll testing.

position; allow any additional nystagmus to subside, and then turn the head 90° quickly to the opposite side and observe for nystagmus. Geotropic nystagmus is more commonly seen, with very intense horizontal nystagmus beating toward the ear that is down, which is the affected side. After rolling to the unaffected side, there is less intense horizontal nystagmus observed but now changing sides and again beating toward the ear that is down. Apogeotropic nystagmus is less commonly seen, beating toward the upper ear, also changing direction when rolled to the unaffected side, again beating toward the upper ear. It is theorized the debris is located close to the ampulla of the semicircular canal or is adherent to the ampulla as in cupulolithiasis (see **Fig. 3**).

TREATMENT OF BENIGN PAROXYSMAL POSITIONAL VERTIGO

The spontaneous rate of symptomatic resolution of BPPV has been shown to range from 20% to 80% at 1 month versus 35% to 50% by 3 months of follow-up in a recent Cochrane report.[4] As a result, the American Academy of Otolaryngology's (AAO) 2017 clinical practice guidelines support observation as an option for the management of posterior and lateral canal BPPV in some patients, although the panel was strongly in favor of treatment with canalith repositioning maneuver (CRP) because of the value of the expedited time of vertigo resolution. It was thought that observation may not be suitable for patients who are older or at high risk of falling, for example, those with pre-existing balance disorders.[4]

Vestibular suppressant medications, such as antihistamines (Meclizine, dimenhydrinate [Dramamine]), anticholinergics (scopolamine [Transderm Scop]), or benzodiazepines (diazepam [Valium]), should not be routinely prescribed to treat BPPV.[4] They have not been shown to be effective and may actually prolong recovery. In addition, potential harmful side effects include a decrease in cognitive function as well as adverse effects on gastrointestinal motility, urinary retention, and vision. These adverse effects are increased in the elderly, which is the population most affected by BPPV,[6] also contributing to dry mouth or changes in vision. The exception would be the potential for short-term use in extremely symptomatic patients.

It stands to reason that because BPPV is a mechanical condition that it would require a mechanical treatment for resolution, but it is only as recently as the 1980s that Brandt and Daroff[11] developed a series of exercises for the treatment of posterior canal BPPV for habituation, followed by Alain Semont and colleagues[12] with the Semont (or liberatory) maneuver and the CRP, or the Epley maneuver developed by John Epley[13] for freeing adhered otoconia on the cupula (cupulolithiasis) or by moving free-floating debris (canalithiasis) from the involved semicircular canal back into the vestibule.[3]

One of the newer positioning maneuvers is the half somersault or Colorado maneuver.[14] Although it has not been as vigorously studied as the other maneuvers, it is readily described when researching BPPV on the Internet and patients often ask about it.

Although originally designed to be performed by a medical practitioner, both the Epley maneuver and Semont maneuver may be done by patients at home and have been shown to be more effective than Brandt-Daroff exercises (64% vs 23% improvement).[4]

The barbecue roll maneuver was initially described in 1996 for the treatment of lateral semicircular canal BPPV,[3,4,10] followed by the Gufoni maneuver in 1998.[3,14]

The number of CRPs needed for resolution of symptoms varies, with some practitioners performing 1 cycle during the initial treatment and others repeating the maneuvers several times until Dix-Hallpike converts to negative.[3,4]

Reviews have concluded that 32% to 90% of patients cleared with the first treatment, 40% to 100% after the second treatment, 67% to 98% after the third treatment, 87% to 100% after the fourth treatment, and 100% in studies in which 5 treatments were received.[4,15,16]

Potential side effects of CRP occur in about 12% of treated patients, including a sense of falling within 30 minutes after the maneuver, postural instability that may last up to 24 hours following the maneuver, nausea, vomiting, fainting, or conversion to lateral canal BPPV, which occurs in about 6% to 7% of treated patients.[3,4]

TREATMENT OF POSTERIOR CANAL BENIGN PAROXYSMAL POSITIONAL VERTIGO

Brandt-Daroff exercises are one type of vestibular rehabilitation (VR), specifically designed to treat BPPV by habituation. Although they have been found to be more effective than sham treatment, they have been found to be less effective than CRP. A Cochrane review supported using CRP for initial treatment but found that VR could be useful to aid in long-term function recovery[4] (**Fig. 4**).

- The patient begins by sitting in the upright position.
- The patient lies down to the affected side, with the head tilted up 45°. The original instructions are to move quickly, but it can be done slowly to be better tolerated by patients. The patient remains in that position until the vertigo resolves, plus another 10 to 20 seconds (see **Fig. 4**A)

The patient sits up and remains in the upright position until the vertigo resolves.

- The patient lies down to the opposite side, with the head tilted up 45°, and remains in that position until the vertigo resolves, plus another 10 to 20 seconds, then return to the upright position (see **Fig. 4**B).

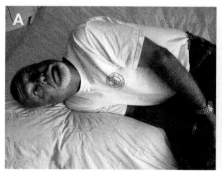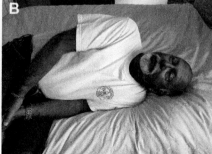

Fig. 4. (*A, B*) Brandt-Daroff habituation exercises.

- The patient repeats maneuvers, alternating sides, working up to 10 repetitions as tolerated, twice a day. Recovery has been reported within 3 to 14 days of treatment.[13,16]

Canalith Repositioning Maneuver (Epley Maneuver)

- Place the patient sitting in the upright position with the head turned 45° toward the affected ear as identified with Dix-Hallpike testing[3,4,13] (**Fig. 5**, right ear). As with the Dix-Hallpike test, eyeglasses should be removed and the patient should be warned that positioning will likely trigger vertigo or nausea but rarely vomiting (see **Fig. 5A**).
- Rapidly lay the patient back to the 20° head-hanging supine position and maintain until vertigo and nystagmus have resolved or at least 20 to 30 seconds (see **Fig. 5B**).
- Turn the patient's head 90° toward the opposite side and hold that position until vertigo and nystagmus have resolved or at least 20 seconds (see **Fig. 5C**).
- Have the patient turn onto his or her side, effectively turning the head another 90°, such that they are looking down at the ground and tucking the chin into the chest. Hold this position for another 20 to 30 seconds or until vertigo and nystagmus have resolved (see **Fig. 5D**).
- Bring the patient into the upright sitting position, holding onto the shoulders as further vertigo resolves.

A 2016 meta-analysis of CRP found that treated patients had a 6.5 times greater chance of improvement in clinical symptoms compared with controls.[4,17] As originally described by Epley,[13] a vibratory device was positioned over the mastoid tip of the affected side during the procedure; but CRP without a device has been

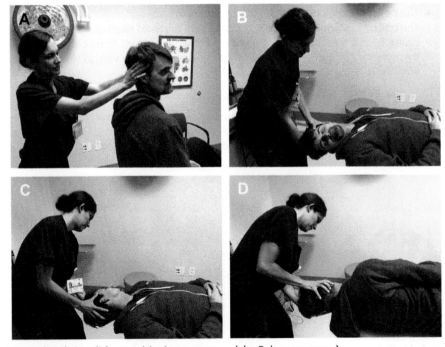

Fig. 5. (A–D) Canalith repositioning maneuver (aka Epley maneuver).

found to be just as effective, although some practitioners will use one in refractory cases.[4] Activity restrictions were commonly prescribed following CRP, including sleeping in the upright position for 48 to 72 hours; sleeping with the treated ear in a dependent position or restricting vertical movement of the head and soft cervical collars have also been used to restrict head movement.[3,13] In a meta-analysis by Devaiah and Andreoli,[18] no effect in outcome was found when comparing groups with restrictions or no restrictions.[4,18] As a result, the AAO's clinical practice guideline BPPV update of 2017 gives a strong recommendation against postprocedural postural restrictions after CRP.[4]

Liberatory Maneuver AKA Semont Maneuver (**Fig. 6** A,B - right ear)

- Place the patient sitting on the examination table with the head turned away from the affected side as identified with Dix-Hallpike testing. Eyeglasses should be removed, and the patient should be warned that vertigo is likely to be triggered by positioning. Advise the patient to keep his or her eyes open during all positioning.
- Quickly move the patient toward the affected side, into the side-lying position with the head turned up and remain in this position until nystagmus has resolved, plus an additional 20 seconds or more.
- Quickly move the patient up and through the sitting position, into the opposite side-lying position, thus, with the head now facing down. Keep the patient in this position until nystagmus has resolved, plus an additional 30 seconds or more.
- Bring the patient up to the sitting position, moving at a normal or slow rate.

A recent Cochrane review showed no difference in effectiveness when comparing the liberatory maneuver with CRP.[4,19]

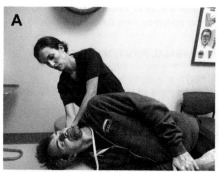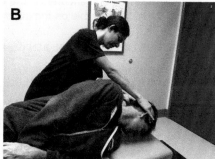

Fig. 6. Liberatory maneuver (aka Semont maneuver).

Half Somersault Maneuver AKA Colorado Maneuver (**Fig. 7**A, B, C, D - right ear)

- This maneuver may be performed at home by patients seated on their knees with arms outstretched to palms on floor in front of them and the head tilted straight up to look at ceiling (see **Fig. 7**A).
- The head is then placed down in a somersault position (see **Fig. 7**B).
- The head is then turned to face the elbow of the affected side (see **Fig. 7**C).
- The head is quickly raised to level of the back, keeping it turned to the side (see **Fig. 7**D).
- The head is fully raised upright.

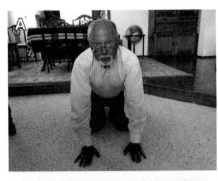
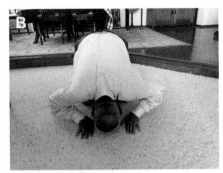
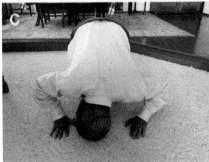
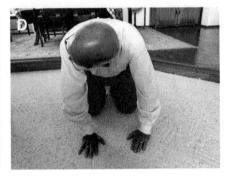

Fig. 7. Half somersault maneuver (aka Colorado maneuver).

    Unlike CRP or the liberatory maneuver, the Colorado maneuver has not been vigorously studied and is not mentioned in the AAO's BPPV 2017 update; but it is included here, as it is readily available on the Internet and patients may ask about it.

TREATMENT OF LATERAL CANAL BENIGN PAROXYSMAL POSITIONAL VERTIGO

Barbecue Roll Maneuver (**Fig. 8**A, B, C - left ear)
    This maneuver is effective for only the geotropic type of lateral canal BPPV.

- Start from either the supine position or the side-lying position of the affected ear. Eyeglasses should be removed and the patient advised that positioning is likely to trigger vertigo.
- Roll the body to the unaffected side (see **Fig. 8**A).
- Continue rolling in the same direction until the patient is prone, with the nose down (see **Fig. 8**B).
- Continue rolling to the supine position (full 360°) and then sit up (see **Fig. 8**C).

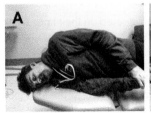
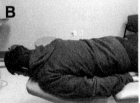
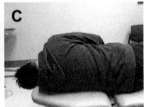

Fig. 8. Barbecue roll maneuver.

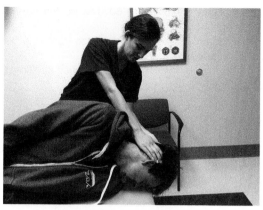

Fig. 9. Gufoni maneuver for geotropic lateral canal BPPV.

Gufoni Maneuver for Geotropic Lateral Canal Benign Paroxysmal Positional Vertigo

- Start from the sitting position. Eyeglasses should be removed, and the patient advised that the position is likely to trigger vertigo[3,4,20] (**Fig. 9**, right ear).
- Move the patient to the straight side-lying position on the noninvolved side for about 30 seconds.
- Quickly turn the patient's head 45° to 60° toward the ground and hold in this position for 1 to 2 minutes (see **Fig. 9**).
- Keeping the head in the turned position, have the patient sit up. Once fully upright, the head is moved back to midline.

Randomized controlled trials (RCTs) have shown both the Gufoni maneuver and the barbecue roll maneuver to be moderately effective for the geotropic type of lateral canal BPPV.[4]

Gufoni Maneuver for Apogeotropic Lateral Canal BPPV (**Fig. 10**-right ear)

- Start from sitting position with eyeglasses removed.
- Move patient to the straight side-lying position on the involved side for about 30 seconds.

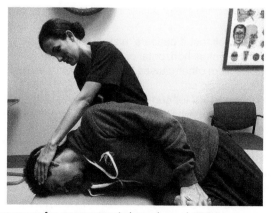

Fig. 10. Gufoni maneuver for apogeotropic lateral canal BPPV.

- Quickly turn the patients' head 45° to 60° toward the ground and hold in this position for 1 to 2 minutes.
  In a variation, the patient's head is moved nose up 45° to 60° and held in this position for 1 to 2 minutes.
- Help the patient sit up, keeping the head in the turned position. Once fully upright, the head is moved back to the midline.

There is only a single RCT with insufficient evidence to support a preferred CRP for the apogeotropic type of lateral canal BPPV.[4]

BENIGN PAROXYSMAL POSITIONAL VERTIGO TREATMENT FOLLOW-UP

It has been recommended that patients should be reassessed within 1 month of the initial evaluation, whether treatment has been observation, VR, or CRP, in order to confirm resolution of symptoms or confirm the diagnosis if symptoms have not resolved.[4] Although most patients are adequately treated with 1 or 2 CRPs (79.4%–92.7%), 5.1% will continue to experience positional vertigo after 2 CRPs and be considered treatment failures.[4,6,16] Follow-up does not need to involve a return visit, especially if patients are symptom free, but could include phone contact or even open-ended follow-up as long as patients are properly educated.[4]

Reevaluation in treatment failures is essential in order to identify and treat possible coexisting vestibular conditions as well as identify possible central nervous system (CNS) disorders, such as multiple sclerosis.[4] For treatment failures confirmed to be BPPV unresponsive to multiple CRPs, either surgical plugging of the involved Posterior Canal or singular neurectomy has a >96% success rate.[4,21]

AMERICAN ACADEMY OF OTOLARYNGOLOGY–HEAD AND NECK SURGERY'S 2017 RECOMMENDATIONS

The AAO–Head and Neck Surgery published an update of their 2008 clinical practice guideline for BPPV in March 2017.[4] This update included recommendations for and against evaluation and treatment options:
Strong recommendation for

- Diagnose posterior canal BPPV when vertigo and torsional, up-beating nystagmus is provoked by the Dix-Hallpike test.
- Treat, or refer to the treating clinician, patients with posterior canal BPPV with a canalith repositioning maneuver.

Recommendation for

- Perform the supine roll test if patients' history is compatible with BPPV and the Dix-Hallpike test provokes horizontal or no nystagmus.
- Differentiate BPPV from other causes of vertigo, dizziness, or imbalance or refer to a clinician who can do so.
- Assess patients with BPPV for comorbidities that may affect management or recovery, such as impaired mobility/balance, CNS disorders, lack of home support, and/or increased risk of falling.
- Reassess patients within 1 month of evaluation and/or treatment to document resolution or persistence of symptoms.
- Evaluate patients, or refer to the clinician, for unresolved BPPV and/or underlying peripheral vestibular or CNS disorders.
- Educate patients regarding the impact of BPPV: safety, potential for recurrence, and the importance of follow-up.

Strong recommendation against

- Postural restrictions should not be recommended following a CRP for posterior canal BPPV.

Recommendation against

- Radiographic imaging should not be used in patients with BPPV in the absence of additional vestibular signs and/or symptoms inconsistent with BPPV that would warrant imaging.
- Vestibular testing should not be used in patients with BPPV in the absence of additional vestibular signs and/or symptoms inconsistent with BPPV that would warrant testing
- Medical therapy, such as antihistamines or benzodiazepines, should not be used routinely for the treatment of BPPV.

Options

- Observation may be offered in lieu of other treatment as the initial management.
- VR, either self-administered or with a clinician, may be offered as treatment.

SUMMARY

BPPV can have a significant impact on the life of patients and is more likely to occur in the older population, already at risk for falls and subsequent injuries. There are multiple treatment options; patients may require second or third treatments, and BPPV often reoccurs. Recurrent BPPV has been measured from 5.0% to 13.5% at the 6-month follow-up, with a rate of recurrence at the 1-year follow-up as high as 10% to 18%. This rate increases over time, possibly up to 36%, even higher in patients with BPPV following head trauma.

At the time of the initial evaluation and treatment discussion, patients should be educated in order to protect themselves from the risk of falls and allowing earlier recognition of recurrent symptoms, thus, allowing earlier treatment by VR or CRP. With proper recognition by patients and clinicians, most cases of BPPV can resolve quickly with effective treatment.

REFERENCES

1. Gray L. Vestibular system: structure and function. Neuroscience online. Chapter 10. McGovern Medical School, University of Texas; 1997.
2. Available at: www.medicalook.com/humananatomy/. Accessed January 5, 2018.
3. Hornibrook J. Review article benign paroxysmal positional vertigo (BPPV): history, pathophysiology, office treatment and future directions. Int J Otolaryngol 2011;2011:835671.
4. Bhattacharyya N, Gubbels S, Schwartz SR, et al. Clinical practice guideline: benign paroxysmal positional vertigo (update). Otolaryngol Head Neck Surg 2017;156(35):S1–47.
5. Nuti D, Masini M, Mandala M. Benign paroxysmal positional vertigo and its variants. Handb Clin Neurol 2016;137:241–56.
6. Neuhauser HK, Leupert T. Vertigo: epidemiologic aspects. Semin Neurol 2009; 29(5):473–81.
7. Parham K, Kuchel GA. A geriatric perspective on benign paroxysmal positional vertigo. J Am Geriatr Soc 2016;64(2):378–85.
8. Balatsouras DG, Koukoutsis G, Aspris A, et al. Benign paroxysmal positional vertigo secondary to mild head trauma. Ann Otol Rhinol Laryngol 2017;126(1):54–60.

9. Dix MR, Hallpike CS. The pathology, symptomatology and diagnosis of certain common disorders of the vestibular system. Ann Otol Rhinol Laryngol 1952;61: 987–1016.

10. Tirelli G, Russolo M. 360-Degree canalith repositioning procedure for the horizontal canal. Otolaryngol Head Neck Surg 2004;131:740–6.

11. Brandt T, Daroff RB. Physical therapy for benign paroxysmal positional vertigo. Arch Otolaryngol 1980;106(8):484–5.

12. Semont A, Freyss G, Vitte E. Curing the BPPV with a liberatory maneuver. Adv Otorhinolaryngol 1988;42:290–3.

13. Epley JM. The canalith repositioning procedure: for treatment of benign paroxysmal positional vertigo. Otolaryngol Head Neck Surg 1992;107(3):399–404.

14. Foster CA, Ponnapan A, Zaccaro K, et al. A comparison of two home exercises for benign paroxysmal positional vertigo: Half Somersault versus Epley Maneuver. Audio/Neurotol Extra 2012;2:16–23.

15. Amor-Dorado JC, Barreira-Fernandez MP, Aran-Gonzalez I, et al. Particle repositioning maneuver versus Brandt-Daroff exercise for treatment of unilateral idiopathic BPPV of the posterior semicircular canal: a randomized prospective clinical trial with short- and long-term outcome. Otol Neurotol 2012;33:1401–7.

16. Tirelli G, Nicastro L, Gatto A, et al. Repeated canalith repositioning procedure in BPPV: effects on recurrence and dizziness prevention. Am J Otolaryngol 2017; 38(1):38–43.

17. Zhang X, Qian X, Lu L, et al. Effects of Semont maneuver on benign paroxysmal positional vertigo: a meta-analysis. Acta Otolaryngol 2017;137(1):63–70.

18. Devaiah AK, Andreoli S. Postmaneuver restrictions in benign paroxysmal positional vertigo: an individual patient data meta-analysis. Otolaryngol Head Neck Surg 2010;142:155–9.

19. Liu Y, Wang W, Zhang AB, et al. Epley and Semont maneuvers for posterior canal benign paroxysmal positional vertigo: a network meta-analysis. Laryngoscope 2016;126(4):951–5.

20. Appiani GC, Catania G, Gagliardi M. A liberatory maneuver for the treatment of horizontal canal paroxysmal positional vertigo. Otol Neurotol 2001;22:66.

21. Hotta S, Imai T, Higashi-Shingai K, et al. Unilateral posterior canal-plugging surgery for intractable bilateral posterior canal-type benign paroxysmal positional vertigo. Auris Nasus Larynx 2017;44(5):540–7.

Vestibular Migraine
Diagnostic Criteria and Treatment Options

Roseanne Krauter, FNP-BC

KEYWORDS

- Vestibular migraine • Vertigo • Anticonvulsants • Beta-blockers
- Tricyclic antidepressants • Dietary modification • Vestibular physical therapy

KEY POINTS

- Vertigo is defined as a false sensation of self-motion or a false sensation that the visual surrounding is spinning or flowing.
- The strict definition of dizziness is a sensation of disturbed spatial awareness.
- Diagnostic criteria for vestibular migraine and probable vestibular migraine have been established by the Bárány Society and the Migraine Classification Subcommittee of the International Headache Society (IHS).
- There is a need for well-designed randomized controls trials and a standardized outcomes measure tool to provide direction in the treatment of vestibular migraine.

INTRODUCTION
History of Vestibular Migraine

Among providers who treat migraine, vertigo has long-been a symptom present in a subset of their patients. Migraine and vertigo are described together throughout the medical literature canon. As long ago as the second century AD, Aretaeus, a Greek physician, describes a type of headache in which "the eyes may move to and fro and the patient is dizzy."[1] Later, a prominent nineteenth century neurologist, Dr Edward Liveing, defines in detail the varied clinical features of migraine, including "epileptic vertigo," in his famous text, *On Megrim, Sick-Headache and Some Allied Disorders: A Contribution to the Pathology of Nerve-Storms.*[2] Dr Liveing reported vertigo to be present in approximately 10% of his patients with migraines; this incidence rate was later confirmed in modern studies.[3] By the 1960s, pediatricians began to recognize the association between paroxysmal vertigo and migraine etiology in children.[4] The 1980s brought about collaboration between neurologists and

Disclosure Statement: The author has no direct financial interest in the subject matter or materials discussed in the following article.
Department of Otolaryngology–Head & Neck Surgery, University of California San Francisco Medical Center, 2380 Sutter Street, 3rd Floor, San Francisco, CA 94115, USA
E-mail address: Roseanne.Krauter@ucsf.edu

Physician Assist Clin 3 (2018) 163–180
https://doi.org/10.1016/j.cpha.2017.11.005
2405-7991/18/ **physicianassistant.theclinics.com**

otolaryngologists that led to published findings regarding large cohorts of patients with both migraine and vestibular symptoms[5–8] and successful treatment of these patients with migraine prophylaxis.[9] However, it would not be until 2012 that a gathering of specialists first defined the terminology and diagnostic criteria for vestibular migraine.[10]

A large swath of terminology (migraine equivalents, migraine-associated vertigo, migraine-associated dizziness, migraine-related vestibulopathy, and migrainous vertigo) has been used interchangeably to describe the same condition. Patients with this condition of many names often present with an unwieldy constellation of symptoms as well. Academic governing bodies recognized the need to provide clinicians with a criteria to accurately and consistently make the diagnosis of vestibular migraine. The Committee for Classification of Vestibular Disorders of the Bárány Society and the Migraine Classification Subcommittee of the International Headache Society (IHS), in a combined effort, established the diagnostic criteria for vestibular migraine.[10] Otologists, neurologists, and vestibular physiologists from the 2 groups convened in 2012 to outline the diagnosis that had been enigmatic to the medical community for centuries.

Diagnostic Criteria

Vestibular migraine and probable vestibular migraine are strictly clinical diagnoses. Making an accurate diagnosis requires attention to detail in history taking. The patient simply stating that he or she feels dizzy is inadequate. Oftentimes patients have difficulty finding the right words to describe their symptoms. True vertigo is defined as a false sensation of self-motion or a false sensation that the visual surrounding is spinning or flowing.[10] The strict definition of dizziness is a sensation of disturbed spatial awareness. Vertigo or dizziness episodes that are spontaneous, positionally triggered, visually induced, or head-motion induced can each be attributable to vestibular migraine or probable vestibular migraine. In addition to the type of vestibular symptoms and potential triggers, clinicians should take note of the duration and frequency of symptoms. The patient needs to have experienced at least 5 episodes of vertigo or dizziness lasting 5 minutes to 72 hours to meet diagnostic criteria. The vestibular symptoms must be either moderate (interfering but not prohibiting daily activities) or severe (inhibiting daily activities) in magnitude.

Vestibular symptoms alone are not sufficient to make the diagnosis of vestibular migraine or probable vestibular migraine. A patient also must present with migraine symptoms along with at least half of their vestibular episodes to have definite or probable vestibular migraine. The migraine features that may accompany vestibular episodes must include one or more of the following: headache, photophobia and phonophobia, and visual aura. The headaches must be consistent with migraine headache and include 2 of the following: unilateral location, pulsating quality, moderate to severe pain intensity, and aggravation with physical activity. Last and most importantly, the constellation of symptoms cannot be explained by another peripheral vestibular disorder or otherwise defined under the International Classification of Headache Disorders (ICHD).

Definite vestibular migraine is differentiated from probable vestibular migraine in that a current or previous diagnosis of migraine with or without aura is required for the former. It is worth noting that making the diagnosis of probable vestibular migraine does not require the presence of headache (**Tables 1** and **2**).

Table 1
Vestibular migraine diagnostic criteria: fulfills all criteria A to D

A.	Vertigo: false sense of self or environmental motion *or* Dizziness: disturbed spatial orientation	Vertigo can be spontaneous, induced by positional changes, visual stimulus, or head motion. Dizziness must be induced by head motion.	≥5 episodes	Last 5 min to 72 h
B.	Current or previous history of migraine diagnosis[11] Unilateral location, pulsating quality, moderate or severe intensity, aggravated by routine physical activity	Either nausea with or without vomiting *and/or* photophobia and phonophobia. With or without visual, sensory, speech, and/or language, motor, brainstem, or retinal aura.	≥5 episodes	Headaches last 4–72 h
C.	At least 1 or more of the following: 1. Migraine headache (see above) 2. Photophobia/ phonophobia 3. Visual aura		Present with 50% of the vestibular episodes	
D.	Not better accounted for by another vestibular or International Classification of Headache Disorders diagnosis			

From Lempert T, Olesen J, Furman J, et al. Vestibular migraine: diagnostic criteria. J Vestib Res 2012;22(4):167–72.

Pathophysiology

The exact pathophysiology of vestibular migraine is not completely understood. Vestibular migraine is considered a migraine variant; therefore, the current hypotheses for migraine mechanisms are generally accepted as the underlying pathophysiology for vestibular migraine. The hypotheses of cortical spreading depression (CSD) and the trigeminovascular pain pathway are the 2 main pillars of migraine pathophysiology. CSD describes a process of a slowly propagating wave of depolarizing neuronal and glial cells. There is a growing body of evidence to support CSD as the underlying mechanism of migraine aura[12–15] and limited indirect evidence that CSD is noxious and may cause headache as well.[16] There is more evidence to support that the sensation of headache and pain are attributable to the trigeminovascular pain pathway.[12,17,18] This process is described as the activation of trigeminal sensory afferents, in response to CSD, which then innervates cranial tissues, including the meninges and their large blood vessels, resulting in pain. The trigeminovascular pain pathway ties into vestibular migraine, as this is the system responsible for innervating the supply of blood to the inner ear and can modulate rapid vasodilation.[19,20] The potential context for vestibular migraine may be that during CSD there is an extracellular release of signals that would then activate trigeminal afferents on cranial blood vessels, thus resulting in a trigeminovascular vasodilation affecting the peripheral vestibular system.[21] This process alone, however, cannot fully explain vestibular migraine and there is likely a multisystem overlap of central vestibular pathways, contributory migraine triggers, such as abnormal sensory input from the inner ear,

Table 2
Probable vestibular migraine diagnostic criteria: fulfills all criteria A to C

A.	Vertigo: false sense of self or environmental motion *or* Dizziness: disturbed spatial orientation	Vertigo can be spontaneous, induced by positional changes, visual stimulus, or head motion. Dizziness must be induced by head motion.	≥5 episodes	Last 5 min to 72 h
B.	Current or previous history of migraine diagnosis[11] Unilateral location, pulsating quality, moderate or severe intensity, aggravated by routine physical activity OR At least 1 or more of the following: 1. Migraine headache (see above) 2 Photophobia/ phonophobia 3. Visual aura	Nausea with or without vomiting *and/or* photophobia and phonophobia. With or without visual, sensory, speech, and/or language, motor, brainstem, or retinal aura.	≥5 episodes Present with 50% of the vestibular episodes	Headaches last 4–72 h
C.	Not better accounted for by another vestibular or International Classification of Headache Disorders diagnosis			

Data from Lempert T, Olesen J, Furman J, et al. Vestibular migraine: diagnostic criteria. J Vestib Res 2012;22(4):167–72.

and premonitory sensory activity. This multisystem overlap is conceptually presented by Furman and colleagues[22] (**Fig. 1**).

Incidence and Demographics

Most medical providers will encounter patients with vertigo at some point in their careers. Dizziness is so common that it accounts for 2.6% of primary care visits in the United States annually.[23] Migraine is another common disorder, and lifetime prevalence ranges from 13% to 16%.[24–27] People with migraine are more likely

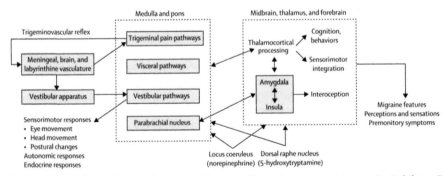

Fig. 1. Potential vestibular migraine pathways. (*From* Furman J, Marcus D, Balaban C. Vestibular migraine: clinical aspects and pathophysiology. Neurology 2013;12(7):710; with permission.)

to experience various forms of episodic vertigo, of which vestibular migraine is only one possible manifestation. Benign paroxysmal positional vertigo, Ménière disease, cerebellar disorders, bilateral vestibular hypofunction, and motion sickness all have an association with migraine and may be easily confused with vestibular migraine. The German National Health Survey conducted a series of telephone interviews to estimate a lifetime prevalence of 1% for definite vestibular migraine (probable vestibular migraine was excluded).[28] If probable vestibular migraine is included with this study's data, the approximate lifetime prevalence increases to 3.2%, making it one of the most common vestibular disorders. To put this into context, the lifetime prevalence of benign paroxysmal positional vertigo is 2.4% and the incidence of Ménière disease is estimated between 15 and 190 per 100,000 population.[29–31]

Vestibular migraine may present at any point in the lifetime. Benign paroxysmal vertigo of childhood is likely an early manifestation of vestibular migraine affecting approximately 2.8% of children.[32] Like other forms of migraine, vestibular migraine affects women more commonly then men.[3]

Making the Diagnosis and Testing

Making the diagnosis of vestibular migraine and probable vestibular migraine is strictly based on the patient's reported symptoms and the exclusion of other possibilities. Allowing adequate time for history taking is imperative to glean the necessary information from the patient. Oftentimes patients will oversimplify when describing attacks or episodes. Definitions of dizziness will vary widely from person to person and the onus is on the medical provider to elicit the details of each patient's vestibular symptoms. Offering descriptive adjectives or phrases, such as "spinning, rocking, feeling 'off,' lightheadedness, feeling as if about to pass out, sense of continued momentum, or floating sensation" can be helpful prompts for symptoms that can be difficult to describe. Taking note of (1) triggering factors, such as rotational movement of the head, visual stimulus, and positional changes; (2) a clear description of the character of vestibular episodes; (3) the duration and frequency of vestibular attacks; and (4) the presence of a migraine history or migraine features with 50% or more of vestibular episodes will allow the provider to assess if these symptoms meet diagnostic criteria for vestibular migraine. The duration of symptoms can be highly variable from patient to patient: 30% lasting minutes, 30% duration of hours, and another 30% persisting for several days.[10] The remaining 10% of patients have attacks lasting seconds that are primarily triggered by positional changes or visual stimulus.

Diagnostic testing to confirm the presence of vestibular migraine is not available currently. Diagnostic testing in this situation is most useful in narrowing the differential or fulfilling the "not better accounted for by another vestibular or ICHD diagnosis" requirement of the vestibular migraine diagnostic criteria. MRI of the brain and internal auditory canal (IAC), computed tomography (CT) of the temporal bone, videonystagmogram (VNG), vestibular-evoked myogenic potentials (VEMP), video head impulse testing (vHIT), rotatory chair testing, and audiogram are all commonly used tests in the evaluation of vertigo.

MRI of the brain and temporal bone is useful for ruling out IAC, cochlear, or intralabyrinthine tumors as well as central causes for vertigo, such as neurodegenerative disorders and cerebellar stroke. In the setting of a routine vertigo workup, a temporal bone CT is most useful in evaluating for superior semicircular canal dehiscence. A standard VNG includes a battery of tests evaluating the function of the vestibular portions of the inner ear and brain. Infrared goggles are used to track nystagmus provoked by visual stimulus, positional changes, and caloric (temperature) stimulation of the labyrinth. In vestibular migraine, VNG test results are typically unremarkable, although a low-level positional nystagmus is common.[33] Anecdotally, in otology practice, it commonly noticed that patients with vestibular migraine have particular difficulty completing VNG testing. Sometimes this noninvasive test is intolerable to migraineurs because of nausea and vomiting, and otologists will use this as an indicator for the diagnosis of vestibular migraine.

VEMP testing is a neurophysiologic evaluation of the utricle and saccule, portions of the inner ear that sense linear motion. Sound stimulus is used to activate the utricle and saccule, which then signals the vestibular nuclei in the brain stem, which activates a reflex in the sternocleidomastoid and occular muscles. There is little evidence to support abnormal VEMP outcomes in patients with vestibular migraine. Only cervical VEMP is discussed, given the scope of this article. Several studies found that abnormal cervical VEMP results were more common in patients with vestibular migraine compared with patients with migraine alone and compared with healthy controls.[34–37] However, other studies, including a retrospective of 39 patients with vestibular migraine and a prospective of 38 women with vestibular migraine, both in comparison with healthy controls, found no significant difference in VEMP latencies and amplitudes.[38–40]

vHIT is used to assess the vestibulo-ocular reflex (VOR). Abnormal vHIT findings are a corrective saccade (shift) in eye movements, seen with quick turns of the head during attempted visual fixation. One retrospective study found 11% of patients with vestibular migraine had abnormal vHIT findings; however, there were no exclusion criteria for patients who may have had a prior peripheral vestibular hypofunction but who had not centrally compensated.[34] This same study noted 19% of patients with vestibular migraine in this cohort had abnormal caloric testing, which again points to a preexisting peripheral vestibular hypofunction clouding the data. A small prospective study showed 8% of patients with vestibular migraine had abnormal vHIT results; however, all 3 of these patients had abnormal caloric testing on VNG as well.[41]

Rotatory chair test also looks at the VOR; one group found a very slight gain in vestibulo-ocular reflexes in patients with vestibular migraine, but it did not statistically differ from patients with classic migraine alone.[42] Audiogram findings are typically normal in patients with vestibular migraine alone; however, audiogram is useful for ruling out peripheral vestibular disorders, such as Ménière disease, mobile third window, and IAC tumors.

TREATMENT

There is a lack of strong evidence to direct treatment choices for vestibular migraine. A Cochrane review completed in 2015 could not identify any well-designed randomized control trials from which to draw conclusions about optimal vestibular migraine treatment.[43] Providers have instead relied on traditional migraine therapy recommendations, given the suspected similarities in underlying pathophysiology.

Making a decision between an abortive versus a prophylactic medication regimen is based on the frequency of vestibular attacks. There are no studies directly comparing the effectiveness of abortive versus prophylactic medication. When looking at individual studies evaluating the effectiveness of abortive medication in vestibular migraine, the evidence shows marginal benefit. Larger studies evaluating the use of prophylactic treatment found benefit; however, each of these studies grouped together the outcomes of several medications and some patients underwent a multistep therapeutic approach, including dietary modification, lifestyle modification, and vestibular physical therapy. There are very few studies testing single medication prophylactic therapy against placebo-controlled groups for vestibular migraine.

In a retrospective chart review including multiple medications (anticonvulsants, tricyclic antidepressants, beta-blockers, valproic acid) and nonpharmacologic treatment (vestibular physical therapy, self-care techniques, and diet modification), 80% of patients receiving treatment with prophylactic medication over 6 months reported a decrease in frequency of vestibular attacks, with 65% of patients noting a decrease in duration of episodes, and 68% of patients experiencing a decrease in intensity of vertigo or dizziness.[44] Patients taking prophylactic medications also showed improvement in nonvestibular symptoms, such as headache, photophobia, phonophobia, nausea, vomiting, and visual and auditory symptoms. A second retrospective review that culled data from the medical records of patients with vestibular migraine taking a combination of prophylactic medications, such as benzodiazepines and selective serotonin reuptake inhibitors, in addition to diet and lifestyle modifications, cited a surprising 92% success rate of resolution or substantial improvement in vestibular symptoms with this combination therapy.[45] Although this study was completed 15 years before the establishment of the vestibular migraine diagnostic criteria, the inclusion criteria were very similar to the current diagnostic criteria and included a thorough evaluation to rule out other peripheral vestibular causes.

There was one prospective observational study of 36 patients who had recurrent vertiginous spells, which was also completed before the establishment of the vestibular migraine diagnostic criteria.[46] The inclusion criteria for this study were very similar to the vestibular migraine diagnostic criteria, but omitted a strict definition of vertigo and dizziness. This study included the use of beta-blockers, tricyclic antidepressants, and clonazepam. Medications were administered for 6 to 42 months and there was a complete resolution of vestibular episodes in 57.6% of subjects, with frequency of vestibular attacks reduced by more than half in 24.2% of study participants.

ABORTIVE THERAPY
Triptans

Two well-constructed studies have been completed for the evaluation of triptans in the use of vestibular migraine. A randomized, double-blind, placebo-controlled, crossover-after-1-attack trial used 2.5 to 5.0 mg orally administered zolmitriptan as needed for acute migrainous vertigo.[47] Subjects taking zolmitriptan 5 mg with vestibular migraine attacks experienced abatement of symptoms in 38% of vestibular attacks; however, the placebo group also had a positive effect in 22% of vestibular attacks. Interestingly, zolmitriptan was less effective than placebo for headache response. Unfortunately, the findings of this study are inconclusive because of the large confidence intervals and the small number of patients recruited (10) with only 17 reported attacks.

A second double-blind, randomized, placebo-controlled study selected 25 patients with migraine with or without the presence of dizziness and the measured effect of rizatriptan on motion sickness induced by a complex vestibular stimulus.[48] Rizatriptan reduced motion sickness in 86% of subjects and this was a statistically significant finding. Although this study does not directly address vertigo attacks in vestibular migraine, there is an indication of potential benefit from rizatriptan use in patients with migraine who experience motion sickness.

PROPHYLACTIC
Anticonvulsants

Topiramate is a medication commonly used to treat seizure and various forms of migraine. Baier and colleagues[44] included 6 patients taking topiramate in their retrospective review cohort of 100 patients. The evidence found from this study supports the use of prophylactic medication for patients with vestibular migraine; however, results of the use of topiramate alone were not reported.

A second retrospective chart review evaluated the effects of topiramate alone.[49] For 17 patients who failed to gain improvement in vestibular symptoms following cessation of caffeine, a 50-mg to 100-mg titration of topiramate was administered. Only 25% of patients with vestibular migraine experienced relief in their symptoms with the use of this medication.

Acetazolamide is commonly used to treat seizures, altitude sickness, and migraine. In a retrospective study, without negative controls or blinding, 39 patients with vestibular migraine took 500 mg per day of acetazolamide as the sole therapeutic agent.[50] Instead of measuring the percentage of patients who gained benefit from acetazolamide, the average frequency and severity of vertigo and headache episodes cumulatively in the patient cohort were measured as the treatment outcome. The frequency of vertigo reduced from 3.9 to 1.4 episodes per month, vertigo severity (determined by visual analog scale) reduced from 5.6 to 2.2, headache frequency reduced from 4.3 to 2.8 per month, and headache severity reduced from 6.2 to 4.1. With the use of acetazolamide 500 mg daily, patients with vestibular migraine experienced a reduction in both the severity and frequency of vertigo and headaches.

Lamotrigine 50 to 150 mg was taken by 3 patients in the study by Baier and colleagues[44] that showed improvement in 80% of patients taking prophylactic therapy. Direct outcome measures of lamotrigine alone were evaluated in a retrospective observational study of 19 patients suffering from migraine and migraine-related vertigo.[51] Patients were given a lamotrigine titration to 100 mg per day in a single dose and were followed for 4 months. The average vertigo frequency per month was significantly reduced from 18.1 to 5.4 and the average headache frequency per month was reduced from 8.7 to 4.4, but the headache findings did not reach statistical significance.

Tricyclic Antidepressants

Amitriptyline was given to a small number of patients in a wide dosage range in 2 of the large retrospective studies looking at prophylactic migraine treatment.[44,46] Patients taking amitriptyline accounted for 42% of the cohort in the retrospective chart review by Johnson[45] that cited 92% success rate with prophylactic medication. Currently there are no studies looking at amitriptyline as a single therapeutic agent for vestibular migraine.

In the previously mentioned retrospective chart review by Mikulec and colleagues,[49] nortriptyline was used as an alternative to topiramate for patients with persistent vestibular symptoms following caffeine cessation. A titration from 25 to 75 mg nortriptyline was given to 22 patients (5 of whom had switched from the topiramate arm) and

46% to 57% of patients reported a reduction in dizziness. This finding was statistically significant.

Beta-Blockers

Currently there are no published studies evaluating the use of metoprolol or propranolol individually. There is an ongoing multicenter, double-blind, placebo-controlled trial on the prophylactic treatment of vestibular migraine with metoprolol 95 mg per day (PROVEMIG-trial).[52] Recruitment was slated to be completed in late 2016.

In the 3 large retrospective studies citing an 80% to 97% success rate with prophylactic treatment, beta-blockers accounted for 30% to 66% of the patient cohort.[44–46] However, it should be noted that these data are clouded, as they include both monotherapy and combination therapy with beta-blockers and other antimigraine pharmaceuticals.

Valproic Acid

One randomized, double-blind, placebo-controlled with crossover design study, published in 1993, looked at the vestibulo-ocular responses in 12 patients with migraine without aura. The VOR measurements were normal in 58% of the cohort despite reported symptoms of vertigo and dizziness; which helped to exclude peripheral vestibular etiologies. These patients then took 600 mg valproic acid per day for an 8-week period and there was no change in vestibular complaints compared with patients who received placebo; however, there was a 67% reduction in headache.[53]

Other Pharmaceuticals

Benzodiazepines, including clonazepam, alprazolam, lorazepam, and prazepam, were used alone and as adjuvant therapy for vestibular migraine in several retrospective reviews showing improvement in vestibular migraine.[45,46] Currently there are no published studies evaluating the use of benzodiazepines individually in vestibular migraine.

Selective serotonin reuptake inhibitors (sertraline, fluoxetine, or paroxetine) were used in 6 of the patients in the Johnson[42] retrospective chart review showing benefit with prophylactic medication. Currently there are no published studies evaluating the use of selective serotonin reuptake inhibitors individually in vestibular migraine.

Supplements

Magnesium (100–500 mg) and butterbur (50–150 mg) were used in 3 and 4 patients, respectively, included in the retrospective study by Baier and colleagues[44] showing potential effectiveness in patients with vestibular migraine. A meta-analysis of randomized controlled trials showed that oral magnesium significantly reduced the intensity and frequency of classic migraine.[54] Similarly, studies evaluating butterbur and classic migraine show efficacy in prevention of headache.[55–57] Like magnesium and butterbur, riboflavin (vitamin B2) has not been evaluated for vestibular migraine specifically; however, the use of riboflavin treatment in migraine is well accepted for significant reduction in headache frequency.[58–60]

NONPHARMACOLOGIC
Vestibular Physical Therapy

There are several studies that have evaluated the effectiveness of vestibular physical therapy in the setting of vestibular migraine. In the retrospective study by Baier and colleagues,[44] 26 patients were treated with conservative therapy, which included vestibular physical therapy, without the use of prophylactic medication. Forty-six percent of these patients noted a decrease in intensity and frequency of vestibular episodes and 42% also noted a shorter duration of vertigo attacks. It is worth highlighting, however, that the findings were statistically significant only with regard to reduced intensity of vestibular attacks. In this retrospective study, there was no improvement in accompanying migraine symptoms, such as photophobia, phonophobia, and visual and auditory symptoms following nonpharmacologic therapy.

Two additional studies evaluated the efficacy of vestibular physical therapy in vestibular migraine when treated concurrently with a variety of prophylactic migraine medications. A study gleaning data from 28 patients with vestibular migraine completing an inpatient vestibular rehabilitation program found significant improvement in headache with coincident improvement in dizziness and psychological variables following vestibular rehabilitation.[61] However, it is unclear if this outcome is secondary to the vestibular physical therapy, the pharmacologic treatment, or a combination of the two.

An observational study looked at 20 patients with vestibular migraine with significant daily vestibular symptoms who completed a 9-week outpatient vestibular rehabilitation program.[62] Outcomes were measured by validated patient questionnaires and objective testing. The patients with vestibular migraine benefited from rehabilitation; however, these results are clouded by the concurrent use of migraine medications.

Self-Care Techniques

Sixty-one percent of patients with vestibular migraine have cited stress, both mental and physical, as a trigger for vestibular episodes.[43] Recommendations for avoidance of migraine triggers, stress reduction, regular sleep patterns, aerobic exercise, and referral to psychologists for stress reduction are common considerations in the treatment of vestibular migraine.[44,46]

Diet Modification

Potential dietary triggers are something that many providers who treat migraine are aware of; however, there is only a small body of evidence at this time to support dietary factors as contributory to migraine. Most commonly noted dietary triggers are caffeine, alcohol, and chocolate.[63] A small cohort of patients with vestibular migraine stopped dietary intake of caffeine, aged cheeses, and monosodium glutamate for 4 to 6 weeks.[49] Only 14% of these patients noted significant benefit in vestibular symptoms. In the Johnson[45] retrospective review, dietary changes, including elimination of aspartame, chocolate, caffeine, and alcohol, were recommended to 66% of patients. It was noted that dietary management often took several weeks before a significant improvement in vestibular symptoms was appreciated (**Table 3**).

SUMMARY

Vestibular migraine is a common disorder that most providers will encounter at some point in their career. This condition typically presents with a wide variety of symptoms and can be debilitating to patients. There are no diagnostic tests currently available to confirm the diagnosis; however, testing can be useful for excluding other vestibular disorders. Medical providers must rely on patient-reported symptoms fulfilling

Table 3
Summary of available data for vestibular migraine treatment

Category	Intervention	Dosage	Study Approach	Limitations	Outcome	Reference
Pharmacologic Abortive	*Zolmitriptan*	2.5–5 mg oral	Double-blinded randomized placebo-controlled trial	Large confidence interval. Small patient cohort.	38% of patients had benefit. 22% of patients on placebo had benefit.	Neuhauser et al,[47] 2003
	Rizatriptan	10 mg oral	Double-blinded randomized placebo-controlled trial	Subject inclusion not specific to vestibular migraine.	86% had less motion sickness following pretreatment.	Furman et al,[48] 2011
Prophylactic Anticonvulsant	*Topiramate*	50–100 mg oral	Retrospective chart review	Small subject cohort.	25% of patients showed benefit.	Baier et al,[44] 2009; Mikulec et al,[49] 2012
	Acetazolamide	500 mg per day oral	Retrospective	No blinding. No controls.	Vertigo frequency and severity reduced. Headache frequency and severity reduced.	Çelebisoy et al,[50] 2016
	Lamotrigine	100 mg per day oral	Retrospective observational	Small cohort. Headache outcome did not reach statistical significance.	Vertigo frequency significantly reduced. Headache frequency reduced.	Bisdorff,[51] 2004

(continued on next page)

Table 3
(continued)

Category	Intervention	Dosage	Study Approach	Limitations	Outcome	Reference
Tricyclic antidepressant	*Amitriptyline*	10–100 mg oral	Retrospective, prospective observational	No individual treatment arm evaluating amitriptyline. Patients on amitriptyline only accounted for 4 of 110 patients.	Grouped in with 80%–97% of patients with improvement who were on various types of prophylactic medication.	Baier et al,[44] 2009; Johnson,[45] 1998; Maione,[46] 2006
	Nortriptyline	75 mg oral	Retrospective chart review	Small cohort.	46% of patients had a reduction in symptoms.	Mikulec et al,[49] 2012
Beta-blocker	*Metoprolol*	50–250 mg oral	Retrospective chart review with controls, prospective observational	No individual treatment arm evaluating the effectiveness of metoprolol. Subjects taking metoprolol accounted for 34 of 100 and 2 of 36 of patients.	Grouped in with 80%–97% of patients with improvement who were on various types of prophylactic medication.	Baier et al,[44] 2009; Maione,[46] 2006
	Propranolol	40–240 mg oral	Retrospective chart review with controls, prospective observational, retrospective review	Subjects taking propranolol 15 of 100, 12 of 36, and 28 of 89. In one of the studies VM criteria were not defined at the time to establish diagnosis.	Grouped in with 80%–97% of patients with improvement who were on various types of prophylactic medication.	Baier et al,[44] 2009; Johnson,[45] 1998; Maione,[46] 2006

Other	Valproic acid	300–800 mg oral	Retrospective review with controls	Accounted for 6 of 100 subjects.	Grouped in with 80% of patients with improvement who were on various types of prophylactic medication.	Baier et al,[44] 2009
			Randomized double-blind placebo-controlled with cross over	12 subjects.	No improvement in vestibular symptoms; 8 of 12 subjects had reduced migraine.	Gordon et al,[53] 1993
	Benzodiazepines[a]	Variable	Retrospective review, prospective observational	Accounted for 74 of 89, 11 of 36, 6 of 89 of subjects. VM criteria was not defined at the time to establish diagnosis in one of the studies.	Grouped in with 92%–97% of patients with improvement who were on various types of prophylactic medication, many subjects were taking a multifaceted approach using lifestyle medication or other pharmaceuticals.	Johnson,[45] 1998; Maione,[46] 2006
	SSRIs[b]	Variable	Retrospective review	6 of 89 subjects. VM criteria were not defined at the time to establish diagnosis.	Grouped in with 92% of patients with improvement who were on various types of prophylactic medication, many subjects were taking a multifaceted approach using lifestyle medication or other pharmaceuticals.	Johnson,[45] 1998
Supplements	Magnesium	100–500 mg oral	Retrospective review with controls	3 of 100 subjects.	Grouped in with 80% of patients with improvement who were on various types of prophylactic medication.	Johnson,[45] 1998
	Butter burr	50–150 mg oral	Retrospective review with controls	4 of 100 subjects.	Grouped in with 80% of patients with improvement who were on various types of prophylactic medication.	Baier et al,[44] 2009

(continued on next page)

Table 3
(continued)

Category	Intervention	Dosage	Study Approach	Limitations	Outcome	Reference
Nonpharmacologic	*Vestibular physical therapy*	Inpatient and outpatient therapy	Prospective, retrospective	Small cohorts of 28, 26 of 100, 20, and 24 of 89 subjects. In several of the studies, most subjects were concurrently on prophylactic medication. VM criteria were not defined at the time to establish diagnosis in 1 of the studies.	Statistically significant improved vestibular symptoms. One group noted improvement in headache; however, a second group found no improvement in headache. There was no effect on migraine symptoms for this group that was not on prophylactic medication concurrently.	Baier et al,[44] 2009; Johnson,[45] 1998; Sugaya et al,[61] 2017; Slavin & Ailani,[62] 2017
	Self-care techniques	Variable	Retrospective chart review with controls and retrospective review	Small cohorts of patients 12 of 100 and 8 of 89. VM criteria were not defined at the time to establish diagnosis in 1 of the studies.	These patients were not on concurrent prophylactic medications; however, the results were grouped in with 80%–97% of patients with improvement who were on various types of prophylactic medication.	Baier et al,[44] 2009; Johnson,[45] 1998
	Diet modification	Elimination of aspartame, chocolate, caffeine, alcohol, aged cheeses, and monosodium glutamate	Retrospective chart reviews	In 1 study, patients were also on concurrent medication prophylaxis.	Dietary modification alone was effective for 14%. In the second study, results were grouped in with 80% of patients with improvement who were on various types of prophylactic medication.	Baier et al,[44] 2009; Mikulec et al,[49] 2012

Abbreviation: VM, vestibular migraine.
[a] Clonazepam, lorazepam, alprazolam, prazepam.
[b] Selective serotonin reuptake inhibitors: sertraline, fluoxetine, paroxetine.

the criteria for vestibular migraine and probable vestibular migraine, set forth by the Bárány Society and the IHS.

There is preliminary evidence to support several classes of medication in the treatment of vestibular migraine, including anticonvulsants, tricyclic antidepressants, beta-blockers, and benzodiazepines. Nonpharmacologic interventions, including vestibular physical therapy, self-care techniques, and dietary modification show potential efficacy as well. At this time, there are no definitive treatment recommendations for vestibular migraine. There is a need for well-designed, randomized controlled trials and a standardized outcomes measure tool to provide direction for providers in the treatment of vestibular migraine.

REFERENCES

1. Huppert D, Brandt T. Descriptions of vestibular migraine and Menière's disease in Greek and Chinese antiquity. Cephalalgia 2016;37(4):385–90.
2. Liveing E. On megrim, sick-headache and some allied disorders: a contribution to the pathology of nerve-storms. London: J. and A. Churchill; 1873.
3. Neuhauser H, Leopold M, von Brevern M, et al. The interrelations of migraine, vertigo, and migrainous vertigo. Neurology 2001;56:436–41.
4. Fenichel GM. Migraine as a cause of benign paroxysmal vertigo of childhood. J Pediatr 1967;71:114–5.
5. Kuitzky A, Ziegler DK, Hassanein R. Vertigo, motion sickness and migraine. Headache 1981;21(5):227–31.
6. Kayan A, Hood JD. Neuro-otological manifestations of migraine. Brain 1984; 107(4):1123–42.
7. Kunkel RS. Acephalgic migraine. Headache 1986;26(4):198–201.
8. Harker LA, Raasekh C. Migraine equivalent as a cause of episodic vertigo. Laryngoscope 1988;98(2):160–4.
9. McCann J. Migraines may manifest as vertigo. JAMA 1982;247(7):956–7.
10. Lempert T, Olesen J, Furman J, et al. Vestibular migraine: diagnostic criteria. J Vestib Res 2012;22(4):167–72.
11. Headache Classification Committee of the International Headache Society (IHS). The International Classification of Headache Disorders, 3rd edition (beta version). Cephalalgia 2013;33:629–808.
12. Pietrobon D, Striessnig J. Neurobiology of migraine. Nat Rev Neurosci 2003;4: 386–98.
13. Lauritzen M. Pathophysiology of the migraine aura. The spreading depression theory. Brain 1994;117(1):199–210.
14. Ayata C. Cortical spreading depression triggers migraine attack. Headache 2010;50:725–30.
15. Charles A. Does cortical spreading depression initiate a migraine attack? Maybe not. Headache 2010;50:731–3.
16. Ayata C, Jin H, Kudo C, et al. Suppression of cortical spreading depression in migraine prophylaxis. Ann Neurol 2006;59:652–61.
17. Olesen J, Burstein R, Ashina M, et al. Origin of pain in migraine: evidence for peripheral sensitisation. Lancet Neurol 2009;8:679–90.
18. Levy D. Migraine pain and nociceptor activation—where do we stand? Headache 2010;50:909–16.
19. Vass Z, Dai CF, Steyger PS, et al. Co-localization of the vanilloid capsaicin receptor and substance P in sensory nerve fibers innervating cochlear and vertebrobasilar arteries. Neuroscience 2004;124:919–27.

20. Vass Z, Shore SE, Nuttall AL, et al. Direct evidence of trigeminal innervation of the cochlear blood vessels. Neuroscience 1998;84:559–67.
21. Iadecola C. From CSD to headache: a long and winding road. Nat Med 2002;8: 110–2.
22. Furman J, Marcus D, Balaban C. Vestibular migraine: clinical aspects and pathophysiology. Neurology 2013;12(7):706–15.
23. Sloane PD. Dizziness in primary care. Results from the National Ambulatory Medical Care Survey. J Fam Pract 1989;29:33–8.
24. Breslau N, Davis GC, Andreski P. Migraine, psychiatric disorders, and suicide attempts: an epidemiologic study of young adults. Psychiatry Res 1991;37:11–23.
25. Lipton RB, Stewart WF, Diamond S, et al. Prevalence and burden of migraine in the United States: data from the American migraine study II. Headache 2001; 41:646–57.
26. Edmeads J, Findlay H, Tugwell P. Impact of migraine and tension-type headache on life style, consulting behaviour, and medication use: a Canadian population survey. Can J Neurol Sci 1993;20:131–7.
27. Rasmussen BK, Jensen R, Schroll M, et al. Epidemiology of headache in a general population–a prevalence study. J Clin Epidemiol 1991;44(11):1147–57.
28. Neuhauser HK, Radtke A, von Brevern M, et al. Migrainous vertigo: prevalence and impact on quality of life. Neurology 2006;67(6):1028–33.
29. von Brevern M, Radtke A, Lezius F, et al. Epidemiology of benign paroxysmal positional vertigo: a population based study. J Neurol Neurosurg Psychiatry 2007; 78(7):710–5.
30. Wladislavosky-Waserman P, Facer GW, Mokri B, et al. Meniere's disease: a 30-year epidemiologic and clinical study in Rochester, Mn, 1951-1980. Laryngoscope 1984;94(8):1098–102.
31. Harris JP, Alexander TH. Current-day prevalence of Ménière's syndrome. Audiol Neurootol 2010;15(5):318–22.
32. Abu-Arafeh I, Russell G. Paroxysmal vertigo as a migraine equivalent in children: a population-based study. Cephalalgia 1995;15(1):22–5.
33. Polensek SH, Tusa RJ. Nystagmus during attacks of vestibular migraine: an aid in diagnosis. Audiol Neurootol 2010;15(4):241–6.
34. Kang WS, Lee SH, Yang CJ, et al. Vestibular function tests for vestibular migraine: clinical implication of video head impulse and caloric tests. Front Neurol 2016;7: 166.
35. Baier B, Stieber N, Dieterich M. Vestibular-evoked myogenic potentials in vestibular migraine. J Neurol 2009;256(9):1447–54.
36. Zuniga MG, Janky KL, Schubert MC, et al. Can vestibular-evoked myogenic potentials help differentiate Ménière disease from vestibular migraine? Otolaryngol Head Neck Surg 2012;146(5):788–96.
37. Boldingh MI, Ljøstad U, Mygland A, et al. Vestibular sensitivity in vestibular migraine: VEMPs and motion sickness susceptibility. Cephalalgia 2011;31(11): 1211–9.
38. Zaleski A, Bogle J, Starling A, et al. Vestibular evoked myogenic potentials in patients with vestibular migraine. Otol Neurotol 2015;36(2):295–302.
39. Kim CH, Jang MU, Choi HC, et al. Subclinical vestibular dysfunction in migraine patients: a preliminary study of ocular and rectified cervical vestibular evoked myogenic potentials. J Headache Pain 2015;16:93.
40. Taylor RL, Zagami AS, Gibson WP, et al. Vestibular evoked myogenic potentials to sound and vibration: characteristics in vestibular migraine that enable separation from Meniere's disease. Cephalalgia 2010;32(3):213–25.

41. Yoo MH, Kim SH, Lee JY, et al. Results of video head impulse and caloric tests in 36 patients with vestibular migraine and 23 patients with vestibular neuritis: a preliminary report. Clin Otolaryngol 2016;41:813–7.

42. Jeong SH, Oh SY, Kim HJ, et al. Vestibular dysfunction in migraine: the effects of associated vertigo and motion sickness. J Neurol 2010;257(6):905–12.

43. Maldonado FM, Birdi JS, Irving GJ, et al. Pharmacological agents for the prevention of vestibular migraine. Cochrane Database Syst Rev 2015;(6):CD010600.

44. Baier B, Winkenwerder E, Dieterich M. "Vestibular migraine": effects of prophylactic therapy with various drugs. A retrospective study. J Neurol 2009;256(3): 436–42.

45. Johnson GD. Medical management of migraine-related dizziness and vertigo. Laryngoscope 1998;108(2):1–28.

46. Maione A. Migraine-related vertigo: diagnostic criteria and prophylactic treatment. Laryngoscope 2006;116:1782–6.

47. Neuhauser H, Radtke A, von Brevern M, et al. Zolmitriptan for treatment of migrainous vertigo: a pilot randomized placebo-controlled trial. Neurology 2003;60(5):882–3.

48. Furman JM, Marcus DA, Balaban CD. Rizatriptan reduces vestibular-induced motion sickness in migraineours. J Headache Pain 2011;12(1):81–8.

49. Mikulec AA, Faraji F, Kinsella LJ. Evaluation of the efficacy of caffeine cessation, nortriptyline, and topiramate therapy in vestibular migraine and complex dizziness of unknown etiology. Am J Otolaryngol 2012;33(1):121–7.

50. Çelebisoy N, Gökçay F, Karahan C, et al. Acetazolamide in vestibular migraine prophylaxis: a retrospective study. Eur Arch Otorhinolaryngol 2016;273(10): 2947–51.

51. Bisdorff AR. Treatment of migraine related vertigo with lamotrigine: an observational study. Bull Soc Sci Med Grand Duche Luxemb 2004;2:103–8.

52. Kalla R, Teufel J, Feil K, et al. Update on the pharmacotherapy of cerebellar and central vestibular disorders. J Neurol 2016;263(Suppl 1):S24–9.

53. Gordon CR, Kuritzky A, Doweck I, et al. Vestibulo-ocular reflex in migraine patients: the effect of sodium valproate. Headache 1993;33:129–32.

54. Chiu HY, Yeh TH, Huang YC, et al. Effects of intravenous and oral magnesium on reducing migraine: a meta-analysis of randomized controlled trials. Pain Physician 2016;19(1):E97–112.

55. Grossmann M, Schmidramsl H. An extract of *Petasites hybridus* is effective in the prophylaxis of migraine. Int J Clin Pharmacol Ther 2001;38(9):430–5.

56. Diener HC, Rahlfs VW, Danesch U. The first placebo-controlled trial of a special butterbur root extract for the prevention of migraine: reanalysis of efficacy criteria. Eur Neurol 2004;51(2):89–97.

57. Lipton RB, Göbel H, Einhäupl KM, et al. *Petasites hybridus* root (butterbur) is an effective preventive treatment for migraine. Neurology 2004;63(12):2240–4.

58. Schoenen J, Jacquy J, Lenaerts M. Effectiveness of high-dose riboflavin in migraine prophylaxis. A randomized controlled trial. Neurology 1998;50(2): 466–70.

59. Sandor PS, Afra J, Ambrosini A, et al. Prophylactic treatment of migraine with beta-blockers and riboflavin: differential effects on the intensity dependence of auditory evoked cortical potentials. Headache 2000;40:30–5.

60. Boehnke C, Reuter U, Flach U, et al. High-dose riboflavin treatment is efficacious in migraine prophylaxis: an open study in a tertiary care centre. Eur J Neurol 2004;11(7):475–7.

61. Sugaya N, Arai M, Goto F. Is the headache in patients with vestibular migraine attenuated by vestibular rehabilitation? Front Neurol 2017;8:124.
62. Vitkovic J, Winoto A, Rance G, et al. Vestibular rehabilitation outcomes in those with and without vestibular migraine. J Neurol 2013;12:3039–48.
63. Slavin M, Ailani J. A clinical approach to addressing diet with migraine patients. Curr Neurol Neurosci Rep 2017;17(2):17.

"Sinus" Headaches
Sinusitis Versus Migraine

Kimberly J.T. Lakhan, DHSc, MPAS, PA-C[a,b,]*

KEYWORDS

- Sinusitis • Rhinosinusitis • Sinus pain • Sinus headache • Facial pain • Migraine
- Trigeminocervical complex

KEY POINTS

- Viruses, not bacteria, are by far the most common cause of acute rhinosinusitis, accounting for most (90%–98%) acute sinus infections.
- There is significant overlap between viral and acute bacterial rhinosinusitis (ABRS), and chronic rhinosinusitis (CRS) and migraine.
- Antibiotics should not be used unless IDSA criteria for ABRS are met; topical steroid nasal sprays and nasal saline irrigations are the mainstay of CRS treatment; triptans should be considered when migraine is suspected.
- Sinus CT scans are helpful if patients are not getting better, or if symptoms continue to recur; however, "sinus" migraine and sinus disease can be comorbid conditions.
- Migraine should be strongly considered in patients with chronic and recurrent "sinus" headache who complain of sinus pain/pressure and nasal congestion, especially when other findings (eg, endoscopy, CT) are lacking or symptoms do not improve with traditional sinus modalities.

"SINUS" AS A PRIMARY COMPLAINT

"Sinus" is a vexing problem for family medicine and otolaryngology practitioners alike. Approximately 30 million people per year annually for the past decade are affected with sinus symptoms in the United States.[1,2] This ranks sinusitis as one of the nation's top five most common health care complaints according to the Mayo Clinic Proceedings,[3] with a direct annual health care cost of $6.9 to 9.9 billion that stems mainly from ambulatory and emergency department services.[4] Annual medication costs for sinusitis were estimated at between $1547 and $2700 USD per patient,[5] with more than one in five antibiotics prescribed in adults for sinusitis, making it one of the top five most

Disclosure Statement: No disclosures.
[a] Department of Physician Assistant Studies, The College of St. Scholastica, 940 Woodland Avenue, Duluth, MN 55812, USA; [b] Department of Otolaryngology, Essentia Health-Duluth Clinic, 502 East 2nd Street, Duluth, MN 55805, USA
* 940 Woodland Avenue, Duluth, MN 55812.
E-mail address: klakhan@css.edu

Physician Assist Clin 3 (2018) 181–192
https://doi.org/10.1016/j.cpha.2017.11.002
physicianassistant.theclinics.com

common diagnosis for which an antibiotic is prescribed.[5,6] In addition, estimates for a total annual economic burden range between \$22 billion and \$64.5 billion USD.[4,5]

Most sinusitis (90%–98%) is caused by the same viruses associated with acute nasopharyngitis (common cold) and acute bronchitis.[2,7] Only 0.5% to 2% of healthy adults and 5% of healthy children develop bacterial superinfections.[7,8] Regardless of the low incidence of true bacterial involvement, and despite the fact that placebo-controlled trials have demonstrated greater than 70% of patients diagnosed with sinusitis show improvement when given placebo,[9] antibiotics are still prescribed at rates upwards of 81% for these patients.[10] To complicate matters further, there is a growing body of evidence that a significant portion of patients with sinus pain/pressure and nasal congestion may have underlying migraine rather than infection as the cause of their symptoms.

SYMPTOMS OF "SINUS" AND DIAGNOSTIC CRITERIA FOR ACUTE BACTERIAL RHINOSINUSITIS

The diagnosis of acute bacterial rhinosinusitis (ABRS) is based on the presence of specific clinical criteria (**Box 1**)[7]; however, these symptoms do not differentiate bacterial from viral sinusitis.[7,11] It is nearly impossible to determine viral infection versus bacterial infection based on clinic symptoms, because of the similar symptomology. Multiple, identical upper respiratory symptoms are associated with both viral and bacterial sinusitis: purulent nasal secretions, maxillary sinus pain, maxillary tooth pain (which is actually uncommon with sinusitis), hyposmia/anosmia, and worsening symptomology after initial improvement form the "short list" of signs and symptoms with some "predictive value," but even these are not an accurate predictor of bacterial involvement.[9]

SYMPTOMS OF "SINUS" AND DIAGNOSTIC CRITERIA FOR CHRONIC RHINOSINUSITIS

The symptoms associated with chronic rhinosinusitis (CRS; sinus symptoms lasting for greater than 12 weeks) are usually the same as the symptoms associated with ABRS.[12] Although CRS symptoms tend to be milder than those of ABRS and may manifest as a single symptom (eg, hyposmia or anosmia), the most common and important symptoms when formulating a differential diagnosis are headache, facial pain/pressure, nasal obstruction, and rhinorrhea.[12]

To confuse and complicate diagnosis and treatment further, many of the same symptoms associated with sinusitis (other than fever) are also associated with sinus headache, making differentiation even more difficult (**Table 1**).[12,13] Additionally,

---

Box 1
Infectious Disease Society of America criteria for ABRS

- Any one of the following clinical symptoms
  - Onset with persistent symptoms or signs compatible with acute rhinosinusitis, lasting for $\geq$10 days without any evidence of clinical improvement;
  - Onset with severe symptoms or signs of high fever ($\geq$39°C [102°F]) and purulent nasal discharge or facial pain lasting for at least 3 to 4 consecutive days at the beginning of illness;
  - Onset with worsening symptoms or signs characterized by the new onset of fever, headache, or increase in nasal discharge following a typical viral upper respiratory infection that lasted 5 to 6 days and were initially improving ("double-sickening").

From Chow AW, Benninger MS, Brook I, et al. IDSA clinical practice guideline for acute bacterial rhinosinusitis in children and adults. Clin Infect Dis 2012;54(8):e72–112.

Table 1
Rhinosinusitis symptoms versus "sinus headache"/migraine symptoms

Rhinosinusitis Symptoms[12]	"Sinus Headache"/Migraine Symptoms[13]
Nasal obstruction	Nasal obstruction
Rhinorrhea/postnasal drainage	Rhinorrhea/postnasal drainage
Facial symptoms (facial congestion, facial pain/pressure/fullness, and headache)	Facial symptoms (orbital edema, facial pain/pressure/fullness, and headache)
Oropharyngeal symptoms (halitosis, dental pain, cough, and ear pain/pressure)	Oropharyngeal symptoms (dental pain, cough, and ear pain/pressure)
Systemic symptoms (fever and fatigue)	Neurologic symptoms (phono/photophobia, gastrointestinal stimulation)
Hyposmia/anosmia	Itchy/watery eyes

From Meltzer EO, Hamilos DL, Hadley JA, et al. Rhinosinusitis: establishing definitions for clinical research and patient care. J Allergy Clin Immunol 2004;114(6):155–212; and Eross E, Dodick D, Eross M. The sinus, allergy and migraine study (SAMS). Headache 2007;47(2):213–24.

headache may be the only symptom in certain patients, such as chronic sphenoiditis, and the headache location may differ contingent on the affected sinuses.[12]

CAUSES OF SINUS PAIN

There are multiple causes for facial and sinus pain/pressure including sinusitis, tension, migraine, cluster, and rebound headaches and temporomandibular joint dysfunction.[12,14–17] The Sinus, Allergy, and Migraine Study (SAMS) found that only 3% of patients met the 2004 Rhinosinusitis Consensus definition for acute rhinosinusitis, whereas 9% of sinus pain was reported as nonclassifiable, 5% as "other," 1% as hemicrania continua, and 1% as cluster (**Fig. 1**).[12,13] In contrast, most of these patients (86%) met the International Headache Society's International Classification of Headache Disorders, 3rd edition (ICHD-3) criteria for migraine and probable migraine headaches (**Box 2**).[13,18]

THE TRIGEMINOCERVICAL COMPLEX

The trigeminocervical complex mediates the pain and symptoms of migraine.[19–21] The trigeminocervical complex is formed in part by the trigeminal caudal nucleus, and

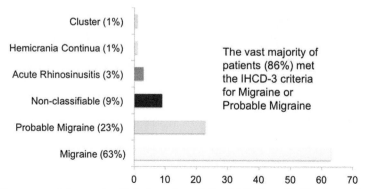

Fig. 1. The causes of sinus pain. (*Data from* Eross E, Dodick D, Erros M. The sinus, allergy and migraine study (SAMS). Headache 2007;47(2):213–24.)

extends from the level of dorsal spinal horn up to the trigeminal nerve distribution in the face and down to C1 and C2 (**Fig. 2**).[21] Stimulation of the superior sagittal sinus, dura mater, and cerebral vessels all in turn trigger the trigeminocervical complex.[21] This complex also receives afferent stimuli converging from the face, teeth, oral mucosa, and the greater occipital nerve, which may account for the migraine triggers emanating from the neck and temporomandibular joint musculature.[21]

Trigeminocervical complex

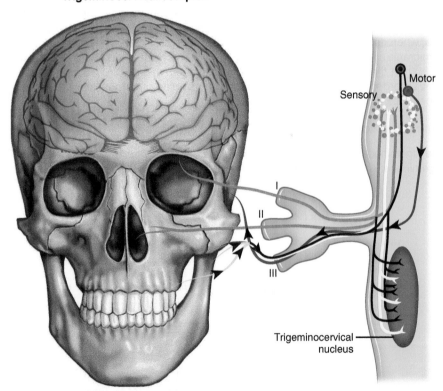

Fig. 2. The trigeminocervical complex.

In a "sinus-like" presentation of migraine, pain can be perceived in the maxillary and ophthalmic regions of the trigeminocervical complex, also causing pain and pressure to be felt in and/or around the eyes and sinuses. Sensitization of the trigeminocervical network can in turn cause nasal congestion with rhinorrhea, itchy nose, periorbital swelling, and lacrimation via stimulation of the parasympathetic fibers during an active migraine.[19,21] Neurologic signs from this heightened parasympathetic stimulation to the head are found during migraine exacerbations in 73% of migraineurs, and are often bilateral.[22]

"SINUS" HEADACHES AS MIGRAINE

Schreiber and colleagues[23] evaluated 2991 "sinus" headache patients for migraine using the ICHD-3 criteria.[18] Of these, 2640 (88%) patients fulfilled the ICHD-3 criteria for either migraine or probable migraine.[18,23] The 2396 patients who met the ICHD-3 criteria for the diagnosis of migraine with or without aura were then screened for sinus symptoms: itchy nose, watery eyes, rhinorrhea, nasal congestion, sinus pain, and sinus pressure (**Fig. 3**).[23] They found that these sinus features of headache where common and likely hid the presence of migraine in patients presenting with common sinus complaints.[23]

Similar findings have been cited in several different studies (**Table 2**).[13,20,23–27] In addition, Cady and colleagues,[28] Ishkanian and colleagues,[29] and Kari and DelGaudio[25] all showed significant reduction in "sinus headache" symptoms when patients were given triptans instead of antibiotics or sinus medications.

COMPUTED TOMOGRAPHY SCANS AND RADIOLOGIC FINDINGS

When it comes to radiographic imaging of the sinuses, computed tomography (CT) provides superior definition of the sinuses and better sensitivity than that of plain radiographs for assessing sinus pathology. This is especially true when the sphenoid and ethmoid sinuses are involved.[30] MRI allows for improved differentiation of soft tissue structures within the sinuses compared with CT; however, its primary role in sinuses disease should be to evaluate suspected tumors or fungal sinusitis because of its tendency to overcall sinus inflammation in asymptomatic patients.[30,31]

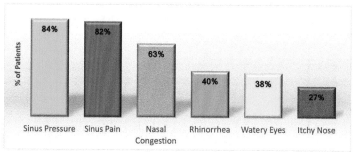

Fig. 3. Sinus symptoms during migraine. (*Data from* Schreiber CP, Hutchinson S, Webster CJ, et al. Prevalence of migraine in patients with a history of self-reported or physician-diagnosed "Sinus" headache. Arch Intern Med 2004;164(16):1769–72.)

Table 2
Summary of studies showing "sinus headache" as migraine

Study, Year	Study Design	Level of Evidence	Number of Subjects	Diagnostic Criteria	Conclusions
Cady,[20] 2002	Prospective	2b	43	ICHD-3 criteria	97% of patients with "sinus headache" had migraine, 3% had tension headache; 73% of moderate or severe pain migraine sufferers experienced improved pain with triptans
Perry et al,[27] 2004	Prospective	2b	36	ICHD-3 criteria	Headache as chief complaint in "sinus" patients, 58% received a migraine diagnosis
Schreiber et al,[23] 2004	Prospective	2b	2991	ICHD-3 criteria	88% of patients had either migraine or probable migraine; most of those with migraine had sinus features/common sinus complaints that likely hid the presence of migraine
Eross et al,[13] 2007	Prospective	1b	100	ICHD-3 criteria	86% of "sinus" patients ICHD-3 criteria for migraine and probable migraine
Mehle & Kremer,[26] 2008	Prospective	2b	35	ICHD-3 criteria	74.3% of "sinus headache" referrals satisfied the criteria for migraine
Kari & DelGaudio,[25] 2008	Prospective	2b	55	ICHD-3 criteria	82% of "sinus headache" referrals responded to empiric triptans
Foroughipour et al,[24] 2011	Prospective	2b	58	ICHD-3 criteria	68% of patients with sinus headache had migraine, 27% had tension-type headache, and only 5% had chronic sinusitis with recurrent acute episodes

Radiologic findings consistent with acute rhinosinusitis on CT include nasal mucosal edema, a sinus air-fluid level, mucosal thickening, and/or complete opacification of an involved sinus.[31] Although acute, traumatic blood in the sinus can also cause an air-fluid level in a sinus, it is usually distinguishable from other secretions by the difference in density on CT.[31] It is also important remember that CT radiologic findings tend to be nonspecific, and thus should not be used routinely when attempting to diagnose acute sinusitis.[30,31] Instead, CT scans should be interpreted in the context of clinical and endoscopic findings.

Up to 40% of asymptomatic adults and more than 80% of adults with acute naso-pharyngitis (the common cold) demonstrate sinus abnormalities on their CT imaging, because the common cold often involves the paranasal sinuses and the nasal passages.[12,31] Meltzer and colleagues[12] reported that these abnormalities were observed in all of the paranasal sinuses of adults and children (with the maxillary sinuses being the most commonly affected), and most of these CT changes resolved spontaneously within 2 weeks of the corresponding cold symptoms resolving.

Ideally, a CT should be used to facilitate the development of a diagnosis and plan for management of recurrent and/or chronic sinusitis, such as defining sinus anatomy before surgery.[30,31] CT findings consistent with CRS usually include mucosal thickening, complete opacification, bone remodeling and thickening caused by osteitis, polyposis, and involvement of the ethmoid sinuses.[31,32]

There are several different CT staging systems used to evaluate radiographic images to determine severity of sinus disease: Lund-Mackay, Jorgensen, Harvard, and Kennedy.[33,34] The Lund-Mackay scoring system has gained most popularity because it is straightforward and easier to apply than other scoring systems. In addition to CT findings, it also includes symptoms, endoscopic findings, and anatomic variations, and a surgical score.[33] It is also worth noting that the radiologic scoring for the Jorgensen staging system does not differ significantly from the Lund-Mackay system.[33] The Lund-Mackay scale is also preferred by the Task Force on Rhinosinusitis.[34]

The Lund-Mackay scale grades the right and left sides independently, looking at the maxillary, anterior ethmoids, posterior ethmoids, sphenoid, and frontal sinuses, and the ostiomeatal complex. Each sinus is scored a 0 (no abnormality), 1 (partial opacification), or 2 (total opacification), whereas the ostiomeatal complex is scored either a 0 or 2 (for presence or absence of disease). Scores range from 0 to 24. Several studies have shown no correlation between Lund-Mackay scores and sinus headache, regardless of migraine status, which suggests that migraine and CRS are likely comorbid conditions (**Table 3**).[26,33–35]

TREATMENT OF ACUTE BACTERIAL RHINOSINUSITIS

The current national recommendations for the treatment of ABRS from the Infectious Disease Society of America (IDSA) were developed in conjunction with other specialties, including experts from otolaryngology.[7] They are to use an antibiotic for patients who have illness symptoms lasting longer than 10 days, with the premise that the longer symptom duration connotes bacterial infection.[2,7,36] At issue, however, is that these recommendations are based on "evidence from RCTs with important limitations (inconsistent results, methodological flaws, indirect, or imprecise) or exceptionally strong evidence from unbiased observational studies."[7]

Once clinical ABRS has been diagnosed, IDSA guidelines[7] recommend that treatment consist of the following[7]:

Table 3
Summary of studies showing correlation between Lund-Mackay scores and "sinus headache"

Study, Year	Study Design	Level of Evidence	Number of Subjects	Diagnostic Criteria	Conclusions
Tarabichi,[35] 2000	Prospective	2b	82	Lund-Mackay score	No association between pain severity and mucosal disease (n = 82)
Jones,[33] 2002	Systematic Review	2a	16 studies	Lund-Mackay score, Jorgensen, and Kennedy	30% of asymptomatic adults showed incidental mucosal changes on CT; percentage even higher in children
Shields et al,[34] 2003	Prospective	2b	51	Lund-Mackay score, Harvard, and Kennedy	No correlation between headache, facial pain, and radiographic abnormalities (n = 51)
Mehle & Kremer,[26] 2008	Prospective	2b	35	Lund-Mackay score	No correlation between Lund-Mackay scores and sinus headache, regardless of migraine status, and suggest that migraine and chronic rhinosinusitis may be comorbid conditions

- Amoxicillin-clavulanate rather than amoxicillin alone is recommended as empiric antimicrobial therapy for ABRS in children (10–14 days) and adults (5–7 days); and
- Doxycycline (100 mg bid) is recommended as an alternative agent in adults who are allergic to penicillin
- Combination therapy with clindamycin plus a third-generation oral cephalosporin (cefixime or cefpodoxime) is recommended in children with a history of non–type I hypersensitivity to penicillin
- Intranasal saline irrigations
- Intranasal corticosteroids

Patients who clinically worsen despite 72 hours or fail to improve after 3 to 5 days of empiric antimicrobial therapy with a first-line agent should be treated with an alternative agent.[7] If the patient's symptoms are still not improving, sinus CT should be considered over MRI, unless fungal involvement or tumor is suspected (because MRI tends to overcall sinus disease).

Antibiotics and medications that should be avoided[7] include macrolides (clarithromycin and azithromycin), because of high rates of resistance among *Streptococcus pneumoniae* (~30%) and azithromycin's poor penetration into the sinuses; trimethoprim-sulfamethoxazole, because of high rates of resistance among *S pneumoniae* and *Haemophilus influenzae* (~30%–40%); and topical and oral decongestants, and antihistamines (unless there are underlying allergies at play), because of limited efficacy.

TREATMENT OF CHRONIC RHINOSINUSITIS

As a chronic inflammatory mucosal disease, CRS cannot be cured for most patients, but it can be managed. The goal of therapy is to control mucosal inflammation and edema, maintain sufficient sinus aeration and drainage, treat colonizing or infecting bacteria (if present), and reduce the overall number of acute superinfections. Nasal saline irrigations and intranasal corticosteroids are the mainstay of treatment.[37–39] In addition, short courses of oral corticosteroids (1–3 weeks) and oral antibiotics (3 weeks) may be beneficial in managing acute exacerbations.[38] The most recent clinical guidelines published by the American Academy of Otolaryngology-Head & Neck Surgery advise against the use of topical or oral antifungals unless the patient has known allergic fungal sinusitis or invasive fungal sinusitis.[37]

TREATMENT OF "SINUS" MIGRAINE

When it comes to the successful treatment and management of acute migraine, experts have long recommended several goals, including consistent and rapid treatment of acute attacks to avoid recurrence, to re-establish the patient's functional abilities, and to curtail the need for back-up/rescue medications (the latter two typically being left to the neurologist or trained family practitioner to mitigate).[16,40] For the acute treatment of migraine, there are two main approaches: nonspecific analgesics, nonsteroidal anti-inflammatory drugs, and aspirin/acetaminophen/caffeine; and migraine-"specific" medications, such as triptans and dihydroergotamine.[16,17,40] Of these, triptans are the most frequently prescribed medication for abortive migraine therapy. There is no evidence to support use of butalbital compounds or opiates in migraine management, and little evidence or support for the use of isometheptene compounds in migraine.[16,17,40]

Other medications, such as sodium valproate, may be used for preventive therapy, but such preventive therapy strategies are best left to the neurologist or trained family practitioner.[16] Several studies successfully used triptans to empirically diagnose migraine in patients presenting with "sinus headache" with response rates upwards of 73%.[20,25,28,29] Based on these findings, it is reasonable to consider a trial with a triptan medication in a patient with "sinus headache," not otherwise explained by history, physical examination, endoscopy, and CT scan, as an appropriate next step for the patient while they await neurology consultation.[16]

SUMMARY

Thirty million people per year for the past decade have been affected with sinus symptoms in the United States, ranking sinusitis as one of the nation's top five most common health care complaints.[1–3] More than one in five antibiotics prescribed in adults are for sinusitis[5,6] despite the fact that viruses, not bacteria, account for most (90%–98%) acute sinus infections.[2,7] There is also significant overlap between viral and ABRS, CRS, and migraine, complicating appropriate diagnosis and treatment. For this reason, antibiotics should not be used unless IDSA criteria for ABRS are met, particularly in this era of antibiotic stewardship.

Sinus CT scans should not be used to diagnose acute rhinosinusitis, given the difficulties with distinguishing viral from bacterial infection on CT radiograms. CT imaging is helpful if patients are not getting better, or if symptoms continue to recur. But it is important to remember that "sinus" migraine and sinus disease can be comorbid conditions. For this reason, migraine should be strongly considered in those patients with chronic and recurrent "sinus" headache who complain of recurrent sinus pain/pressure and nasal congestion, especially when other findings (eg, endoscopy, CT) are lacking or when symptoms do not improve with traditional sinus modalities. Furthermore, triptans may be an effective diagnostic and management tool for acute migraine attacks, and for improving overall function in the patients with "sinus" headache.

REFERENCES

1. National Center for Health Statistics. Summary health statistics: National Health Interview Survey, 2015, Table A-2. 2015. Available at: https://ftp.cdc.gov/pub/Health_Statistics/NCHS/NHIS/SHS/2015_SHS_Table_A-2.pdf. Accessed April 30, 2015.
2. Rosenfeld RM, Andes D, Bhattacharyya N, et al. Clinical practice guideline: adult sinusitis. Otolaryngol Head Neck Surg 2007;137(3 Suppl):S1–31.
3. St Sauver JL, Warner DO, Yawn BP, et al. Why patients visit their doctors: assessing the most prevalent conditions in a defined American population. Mayo Clin Proc 2013;88(1):56–67.
4. Caulley L, Thavorn K, Rudmik L, et al. Direct costs of adult chronic rhinosinusitis by using 4 methods of estimation: results of the US Medical Expenditure Panel Survey. J Allergy Clin Immunol 2015;136(6):1517–22.
5. Smith KA, Orlandi RR, Rudmik L. Cost of adult chronic rhinosinusitis: a systematic review. Laryngoscope 2015;125(7):1547–56.
6. Hsiao CJ, Cherry DK, Beatty PC, et al. National ambulatory medical care survey: 2007 summary. Hyattsville (MD): National Center for Health Statistics; 2010.
7. Chow AW, Benninger MS, Brook I, et al. IDSA clinical practice guideline for acute bacterial rhinosinusitis in children and adults. Clin Infect Dis 2012;54(8):e72–112.
8. Lingard H, Zehetmayer S, Maier M. Bacterial superinfection in upper respiratory tract infections estimated by increases in CRP values: a diagnostic follow-up in primary care. Scand J Prim Health Care 2008;26(4):211–5.

9. Schumann S, Hickner J. PURLs: Patients insist on antibiotics for sinusitis? Here is a good reason to say "no". J Fam Pract 2008;57(7):464–86.

10. Young J, De Sutter A, Merenstein D, et al. Antibiotics for adults with clinically diagnosed acute rhinosinusitis: a meta-analysis of individual patient data. Lancet 2008;371(9616):908–14.

11. Centers for Disease Control and Prevention. Get smart: know when antibiotics work in doctor's offices – Sinus infection (sinusitis). 2015. Available at: https://www.cdc.gov/getsmart/community/for-patients/common-illnesses/sinus-infection.html. Accessed April 22, 2017.

12. Meltzer EO, Hamilos DL, Hadley JA, et al. Rhinosinusitis: establishing definitions for clinical research and patient care. J Allergy Clin Immunol 2004;114(6):155–212.

13. Eross E, Dodick D, Eross M. The sinus, allergy and migraine study (SAMS). Headache 2007;47(2):213–24.

14. Levine H, Setzen M, Holy C. Why the confusion about sinus headache? Otolaryngol Clin North Am 2014;47(2):169–74.

15. Milam B, Ramakrishnan VR. Facial pain and headache. In: Scholes MA, Ramakrishnan VR, editors. ENT secrets. Philadelphia: Elsevier; 2016. p. 46–9.

16. Patel ZM, Setzen M, Poetker DM, et al. Evaluation and management of "sinus headache" in the otolaryngology practice. Otolaryngol Clin North Am 2014;47(2):269–87.

17. Weatherall MW. Headache and facial pain. Medicine 2016;44(8):475–9.

18. Headache Classification Committee of the International Headache Society. The International Classification of Headache Disorders, 3rd edition (beta version). Cephalalgia 2013;33(9):629–808.

19. Buture A, Gooriah R, Nimeri R, et al. Current understanding on pain mechanism in migraine and cluster headache. Anesth Pain Med 2016;6(3):842–7.

20. Cady RK. Distinguishing "sinus headache" from migraine headache. Advanced Studies in Medicine 2002;2(16):582–5.

21. Cortelli P. Migraine and the autonomic nervous system. In: Robertson D, Biaggioni I, editors. Primer on the autonomic nervous system. 3rd edition. London: Academic Press, Elsevier; 2012. p. 545–7.

22. Gupta R, Bhatia MS. A report of cranial autonomic symptoms in migraineurs. Cephalalgia 2007;27(1):22–8.

23. Schreiber CP, Hutchinson S, Webster CJ, et al. Prevalence of migraine in patients with a history of self-reported or physician-diagnosed "sinus" headache. Arch Intern Med 2004;164(16):1769–72.

24. Foroughipour M, Sharifian SM, Shoeibi A, et al. Causes of headache in patients with a primary diagnosis of sinus headache. Eur Arch Otorhinolaryngol 2011;268(11):1593–6.

25. Kari E, DelGaudio JM. Treatment of sinus headache as migraine: the diagnostic utility of triptans. Laryngoscope 2008;118(12):2235–9.

26. Mehle ME, Kremer PS. Sinus CT scan findings in "sinus headache" migraineurs. Headache 2008;48:67–71.

27. Perry BF, Login IS, Kountakis SE. Nonrhinologic headache in a tertiary rhinology practice. Otolaryngol Head Neck Surg 2004;130(4):449–52.

28. Cady RJ, Dodick DW, Levine HL, et al. Sinus headache: a neurology, otolaryngology, allergy and primary care consensus on diagnosis and treatment. Mayo Clin Proc 2005;80(7):908–16.

29. Ishkanian G, Blumenthal H, Webster CJ, et al. Efficacy of sumatriptan tablets in migraineurs self-described or physician-diagnosed as having sinus headache: a randomized, double-blind, placebo-controlled study. Clin Ther 2007;29(1):99–109.

30. Okuyemi KS, Tsue TT. Radiologic imaging in the management of sinusitis. Am Fam Physician 2002;66(10):1882–7.
31. Ramanan RV, Kahn AN. Sinusitis imaging. eMedicine 2016. Available at: http://emedicine.medscape.com/article/384649-overview-a3. Accessed April 22, 2017.
32. Platt MP, Cunnane ME, Curtin HD, et al. Anatomical changes of the ethmoid cavity after endoscopic sinus surgery. Laryngoscope 2008;118(12):2240–4.
33. Jones NS. CT of the paranasal sinuses: a review of the correlation with clinical, surgical and histopathological findings. Clin Otolaryngol 2002;27:11–7.
34. Shields G, Seikaly H, LeBoeuf M, et al. Correlation between facial pain or headache and computed tomography in rhinosinusitis in Canadian and U.S. subjects. Laryngoscope 2003;113:943–5.
35. Tarabichi M. Characteristics of sinus-related pain. Otolaryngol Head Neck Surg 2000;122(6):842–7.
36. Hickner JM, Bartlett JG, Besser RE, et al. Principles of appropriate antibiotic use for acute rhinosinusitis in adults: Background. Ann Intern Med 2001;134:498–505.
37. Rosenfeld RM, Piccirillo JF, Chandrasekhar SS. Clinical practice guideline (update) on adult sinusitis. J Otolaryngol Head Neck Surg 2015;152(2 Suppl):S1–39.
38. Rudmik L, Soler ZM. Medical therapies for adult chronic sinusitis: a systematic review. JAMA 2015;314(9):926–39.
39. Chong LY, Head K, Hopkins C, et al. Intranasal steroids versus placebo or no intervention for chronic rhinosinusitis. Cochrane Database Syst Rev 2016;(4):CD011996.
40. Snow V, Weiss K, Wall EM, et al. Pharmacologic management of acute attacks of migraine and prevention of migraine headache. Ann Intern Med 2002;137(10):840–9.

Pediatric Sleep-Disordered Breathing

William J. Jensen, PA-C, MMS

KEYWORDS

- Pediatric sleep-disordered breathing • Pediatric obstructive sleep apnea • Snoring
- Tonsillectomy • Adenotonsillectomy • Polysomnography • Tonsillar hypertrophy
- ADHD

KEY POINTS

- Pediatric sleep-disordered breathing has replaced throat infections as the predominant indication for adenotonsillectomy in the United States.
- Sleep-disordered breathing has been associated with a negative impact on daytime alertness, emotional lability, attention, school performance, stature/failure to thrive, enuresis, and cardiopulmonary morbidity.
- Sleep-disordered breathing should be considered in the investigation of several common pediatric conditions, including attention-deficit/hyperactivity disorder and other mood disorders, enuresis, and failure to thrive, among others.
- Polysomnography is the gold standard in diagnosis of pediatric obstructive sleep apnea, but its use is not always practical and it is, therefore, not as widespread as might be expected.
- Tonsillectomy shows clear benefits for sleep-disordered breathing and its sequelae as well as for throat infections in the first year after surgery, but longer-term benefits of the surgery are less clear.

INTRODUCTION

Frequently a concerned parent or caregiver may ask a practitioner in a primary care or pediatric office setting, conceivably on a daily basis, "Does my child need tonsils removed?" With more than 500,000 tonsillectomies performed per year, this is a common inquiry.[1] Despite the frequency of this procedure, evidence exists showing the indications for this surgery and the potential benefits are underestimated by health care providers.[1] Although historically tonsils were frequently removed for recurrent infection, today the primary indication for tonsillectomy, with or without adenoidectomy, is sleep-disordered breathing (SDB). The American Academy of Otolaryngology–Head and Neck Surgery (AAO-HNS) has reported that SDB currently accounts for approximately 80% of all adenotonsillectomies (ATs) done in children, whereas throat infections account for approximately 10%.[2] This article reviews SDB, its sequelae, and

Pediatric Otolaryngology, Saint Alphonsus Regional Medical Center, Boise, ID 83704, USA
E-mail address: Bill.Jensen@saintalphonsus.org

Physician Assist Clin 3 (2018) 193–206
https://doi.org/10.1016/j.cpha.2017.12.005
2405-7991/18/© 2017 Elsevier Inc. All rights reserved.

physicianassistant.theclinics.com

the impact on children's health. Current trends in the clinical evaluation of SBD and options for management, namely AT, are discussed.

SLEEP-DISORDERED BREATHING DEFINED

The AAO-HNS defines SDB as a condition that encompasses a spectrum of disorders ranging in severity from snoring to obstructive sleep apnea (OSA) and characterized by "an abnormal respiratory pattern during sleep that includes snoring, mouth breathing, and pauses and gasps." They further delineate disordered breathing in sleep by noting that the prevalence of SDB in children is 10% to 12%, whereas the prevalence of OSA in children is 1% to 3%.[3] Therefore, every child with OSA has SDB, but not every child with SDB has OSA. Specifically identifying where a patient lies on this spectrum from snoring to OSA facilitates the selection of optimal treatment, discussed later. A meta-analysis showed that overall prevalence of snoring was 7% and further demonstrated that SDB is more common among boys than girls, in obese youth, and among African American children.[4]

In *Cummings Pediatric Otolaryngology*,[5] the pathophysiology of SBD is attributed to narrowing of the airway at multiple levels and it is often multifactorial. The primary factors contributing to this narrowing include adenotonsillar hypertrophy, craniofacial abnormalities (eg, micrognathia), laryngeal airway abnormalities (eg, laryngomalacia), and pharyngeal muscular hypotonicity, because it is found in several neuromuscular conditions (eg, cerebral palsy). In syndromic children (eg, Down syndrome), more than 1 of these factors may be encountered, making them a higher-risk population. The authors in Cummings notes that no single factor accounts for all cases, including adenotonsillar hypertrophy. They summarize by stating

> *The current view is that children with OSA have an underlying abnormality of upper airway motor control or tone that, when combined with enlarged tonsils and adenoids, results in dynamic airway obstruction during sleep.*[5]

IMPACT OF SLEEP-DISORDERED BREATHING

SDB is associated with significant negative impact on quality of life (QOL) and overall health. The spectrum of this impact ranges from behavioral to cognitive and from social to cardiopulmonary. Evaluation of SDB should be considered in the following and other related pediatric disorders.[6]

Behavior

Likely the most common behavioral problem associated with SDB is attention-deficit/hyperactivity disorder (ADHD). More specifically, a range of externalizing behavioral issues have been linked to SDB from hyperactivity and inattention to rebelliousness and aggression.[7] The connection between behavior and SDB is strong, with up to one-third of children with loud snoring and/or OSA showing symptoms of ADHD.[8] Furthermore, there has been shown to be improvement in ADHD symptoms after AT indirectly, indicating a connection between the 2 disorders.[9] The sleepiness/hypersomnia resulting from SDB is commonly thought to manifest through inattention and hyperactivity as externalized behaviors in children. This is in contrast to the more familiar symptoms of sleep deprivation seen in adults, such as yawning and drowsiness.[7,10] No concrete mechanisms to explain the association between ADHD and SDB have been found, however. Currently, probable mechanisms are believed intermittent hypoxia and, to a lesser extent, chronic sleep restriction, fragmentation, or some combination of both.[7]

Less frequently, internalizing behaviors, such as depression and anxiety, are associated with SDB. A child's perceived mood, as assessed by caregivers and teachers, has been shown more conclusively to be affected by SDB.[7] The relationship between emotional lability (exaggerated shifts in mood) and SDB has been reinforced by the effectiveness of SDB treatment in stabilizing mood.[6,11]

Cognition

Children with SDB have been shown to perform more poorly on intelligence tests, although association with specific cognitive functions, such as memory, language, and visual perception is minimal.[7] However mild the cognitive impact of SDB may be, when it is combined with more clearly demonstrable neurobehavioral changes, there is a significant effect on school performance. Therefore, screening for SDB should be routinely included in the assessment of children with learning difficulties.[7,12,13]

Enuresis

Of all the sequelae that have been associated with SDB, a unique or perhaps less obvious one is enuresis. Enuresis is common among children, and children with prolonged enuresis have been shown to have lower self-esteem.[14] Several studies have demonstrated the connection between SDB and enuresis, which is present in up to 50% of children with SDB.[1] Approximately 5% to 10% of enuresis seems caused by SDB.[15] One study reported that of possible associated symptoms, such as snoring, mouth breathing, and tonsil size, enuresis had the highest predictive value for SDB.[16] As with other SDB sequelae, AT has been shown to reduce presence of enuresis.[15]

Weight Disorders: Failure to Thrive

SDB has long been associated with growth failure, known as failure to thrive (FTT) in younger children.[17] FTT is seen in 5% to 10% of children in the United States and is defined as either weight per age, which falls below the fifth percentile on multiple occasions, or weight deceleration that crosses 2 major percentile lines on a growth chart. Practically, FTT is characterized by inadequate caloric intake, inadequate caloric absorption, or excessive caloric expenditure. SDB and adenotonsillar hypertrophy are not typically cited as principal causes of growth failure, rather, most cases of FTT are associated with inadequate caloric intake caused by psychosocial/behavior issues.[18] In a literature review on SDB and FTT, 8 studies qualified for review: 6 showed the incidence of FTT in SDB twice what would be expected. These studies also found that AT produced greater than expected weight gain.[19] The impact of SDB on struggles with growth has been ascribed to impaired growth hormone secretion, dysphagia, decreased caloric consumption, and increased caloric expenditure due to nighttime work of breathing.[19–21]

Weight Disorders: Obesity

Results showing reduction in degree of FTT with AT are heartening. The contraposition of this enhanced growth is emerging evidence that AT is also a risk factor for obesity. Consequently, a practitioner recommending AT should educate families on this risk and consider continuous positive airway pressure (CPAP) as first-line treatment of SBD in an obese child.[22] A study in 2013 of 115 patients showed that weight gain after AT is likely age dependent. They found that children 6 years of age or older were more likely to gain weight after surgery. They also found, however, that children less than 6 years of age, even those who were already overweight at time of surgery, did not experience a significant postoperative change in body mass index.[20]

Cariopulmonary Sequelae

Cardiovascular sequelae of SDB in children has perhaps the greatest paucity of research, in contrast to the well-established corollary of cardiovascular impact on adults with OSA. Generally, SDB in all ages has been shown to have a negative effect on blood pressure, cardiac function, and heart rate variability.[23–25] In 2013, Teo and Mitchell[24] performed a systematic review of the effects of pediatric AT on cardiovascular parameters and found only 17 articles meeting their inclusion criteria. They confirmed the negative impact that SBD has on blood pressure, cardiac function, and heart rate variability seems to improve after AT. This systematic review notes, however, that most of the studies included had small sample sizes, lacked utilization of polysomnography (PSG), and lacked control for confounders (such as obesity), which are common in SDB. The investigators also question the noncausal coexistence of SBD in cardiovascular disease.[24] Severe cardiovascular morbidities of SDB, such as heart failure, seem potentially reversible with AT based on the existing body of evidence, but the importance of further studies is clear.[24,26,27]

Quality of Life

QOL has generally been accepted to improve in children after AT.[1] Historically, this understanding was based on the descriptive reports of caregivers, but in recent years this has been objectively demonstrated via validated outcome measures to track perioperative QOL. The first such instrument was developed by De Serres and colleagues—the Obstructive Sleep Disorders-6, which used 6 criteria: physical suffering, sleep disturbance, speech and swallowing difficulties, emotional distress, activity limitations, and caregiver concern. Other instruments following QOL in children with SDB have since emerged, including the Child Health Questionnaire – Parent Form 28, which added measures like self-esteem, family cohesion, and impact on parents both emotionally and on time left for their own personal needs.[28] For example, the state of Oregon requires otolaryngologists requesting prior authorization to perform AT to have had each patient who is insured by state-issued Medicaid to have completed the OSA-18 (**Fig. 1**). The OSA-18, a validated outcome measure, may seem cumbersome to some caregivers but is generally completed without complaint.[29] Many nonrandomized studies (discussed previously) correlated AT with improvement in QOL in patients with SBD, using 1 or more validated scales. The Childhood Adenotonsillectomy Trial, a large, multicenter, randomized, controlled trial, was published in 2013, and, in comparing school-age children who received AT with those randomized to watchful waiting, found that cognitive function did not significantly improve with surgery, but significant improvement was noted in QOL along with symptoms, PSG findings, and behavior.[11]

SLEEP-DISORDERED BREATHING: EVALUATION

A diagnosis of SDB is established through history, physical examination, and evaluation of audio/video recordings, pulse oximetry, and/or PSG.[1]

History

Practitioners should be aware that SDB in children presents differently than in adults. As alluded to previously, children rarely present with a chief complaint of excessive daytime sleepiness but rather with externalizing behaviors of hyperactivity, inattention, and emotional lability. Within the pediatric demographic, some SDB symptoms seem to evolve with increasing age, whereas other symptoms like snoring, pauses, and gasps remain more consistent into adolescence and adulthood[30] (**Table 1**).

OSA18–18 Survey on Quality of Life
Sleep Respiratory Disorder Assessment

Instructions. For each of the questions below, please circle the number that best describes the frequency with which each symptom or problem has occurred within the past four weeks (or since the last survey, if more recently).

	None	Almost None	Few times	Some times	Many times	Most of the time	Every times
Sleep disorders							
For the past 4 wk, how often has your child...							
... snored loudly?	1	2	3	4	5	6	7
... held his or her breath or stopped breathing at night?	1	2	3	4	5	6	7
... choked or had difficulty breathing during sleep?	1	2	3	4	5	6	7
... had agitated sleep or woken up frequently from sleep?	1	2	3	4	5	6	7
Physical distress							
For the past 4 wk, how often has your child...							
... mouth-breathed due to nasal obstruction?	1	2	3	4	5	6	7
... had colds or upper airway infections?	1	2	3	4	5	6	7
... had nasal secretion or runny nose?	1	2	3	4	5	6	7
... had difficulty feeding?	1	2	3	4	5	6	7
Emotional distress							
For the past 4 wk, how often has your child...							
... had mood swings or anger episodes?	1	2	3	4	5	6	7
... behaved aggressively or hyperactively?	1	2	3	4	5	6	7
... had discipline problems?	1	2	3	4	5	6	7
Diurnal problems							
For the past 4 wk, how often has your child...							
... been sleepy or napped excessively during the day?	1	2	3	4	5	6	7
... had difficulty focusing or paying attention?	1	2	3	4	5	6	7
... had difficulty getting up in the morning?	1	2	3	4	5	6	7
Caretaker preoccupation							
For the past 4 wk, how often did the troubles above...							
... leave you worried about your child's overall health?	1	2	3	4	5	6	7
... lead you to believe your child was not breathing well enough?	1	2	3	4	5	6	7
... interfere with you ability to perform your daily duties?	1	2	3	4	5	6	7
... make you feel frustrated?	1	2	3	4	5	6	7

Fig. 1. QOL—sleep respiratory disorder assessment.

The American Academy of Pediatrics (AAP) Clinical Practice Guidelines (CPGs) note that inquiry regarding a history of snoring should be part of routine health care visits and that OSA is unlikely in the absence of snoring. The AAP CPGs on SDB recommend that if a snoring history is elicited, then further questioning into history of other SBD symptoms is warranted.[31]

Furthermore, an index of suspicion for SDB should arise for children with any of the predisposing conditions or disorders listed in **Box 1**. Of particular concern are children with trisomy 21, where the prevalence of OSA is reported to be between 30% and 66% and AT has been shown to decrease the PSG measure of apnea-hypopnea index (AHI) by 51%.[32] *Cummings Pediatric Otolaryngology* explains that the predisposition for SDB in Down syndrome is due to the maxillary hypoplasia, macroglossia, narrow nasopharynx, shortened palate, generalized hypotonia, and a tendency to obesity frequently found in Down syndrome. Furthermore, it explains that as many of the symptoms of SDB (daytime sleepiness, behavioral problems, developmental delay, and pulmonary hypertension) are also common in Down syndrome the diagnosis is often delayed. This issue can be extrapolated to other syndromic children with predisposing factors are present and where the symptoms of SBD are common and this diagnosis overlooked.[2]

Physical Examination

The AAO-HNS published CPGs regarding tonsillectomy, which note that the most common cause of SDB in children is tonsillar and adenoid hypertrophy. Tonsil size

Table 1
Symptoms of sleep-disordered breathing in children by age

Infants, 3–12 mo	Toddlers, 1–3 y	Preschool, 3–5 y	School, 5–18 y
Snoring	Snoring	Snoring	Snoring
Witnessed apnea	Witnessed apnea	Witnessed apnea	Witnessed apnea
Frequent arousals	Frequent arousals	Frequent arousals	Frequent arousals
Mouth breathing	Mouth breathing	Mouth breathing	Mouth breathing
Nocturnal sweating	Nocturnal sweating	Nocturnal sweating	Nocturnal sweating
Nasal congestion	Nasal congestion	Nasal congestion	Nasal congestion
Hyperextended neck	Hyperextended neck	Hyperextended neck	Hyperextended neck
Recurrent AOM/URI	Recurrent AOM/URI	Recurrent AOM/URI	Recurrent AOM/URI
Noisy breathing	Sleep terrors	Drooling	Nightmares
Poor suck	Confusional arousal	Sleep terrors	Sleep talking
Apparent life-threatening event	Irritability	Confusional arousal	Confusional arousal
	Daytime sleepiness	Sleepwalking	Sleep walking
	Restless sleep	Daytime sleepiness/ persistent naps	Daytime sleepiness
Poor day/night cycle		Restless sleep	Restless sleep
Stridor		Enuresis	Enuresis
Breath holding spells		Hyperactivity, inattention	Hyperactivity, inattention
		Difficulty waking up in the morning	Difficulty waking up in the morning
		Drooling	Drooling
		Morning headache	Morning headache
		Sleep in knee-chest position	Insomnia
			Learning difficulties
			Delayed puberty
			Crossbite, malocclusion (class II or III), overcrowding of teeth
			Mood disorder, for example, depression
			DSPS
			Hypertension

From Sinha D, Guilleminault C. Sleep disordered breathing in children. Indian J Med Res 2010;131:311–20; with permission.

is straightforward to identify clinically, using the tonsil grading scale: tonsillar hypertrophy is defined as grade 3+ or 4+ (**Fig. 2**, **Table 2**). The CPGs further note that tonsil size alone does not correlate with degree of SDB, but that combined volume of adenoid and tonsil tissue correlates more closely.[1] In children with symptoms of SDB, tonsil size should be evaluated, in conjunction with a thorough nasal examination, assessment of relative size of the airway, and attention to any craniofacial abnormalities.[33]

Diagnosis with Polysomnography

Obtaining a thorough history and physical examination is important and can indicate to clinicians the impact SDB may be having on a child's life; however, history and physical examination alone are inadequate to reliably diagnose SDB or OSA in children.[3] In addition to history and physical examination findings, audio/visual taping, pulse oximetry, and full-night PSG are used as an adjunct in the diagnosis of SDB.

Box 1
Predisposing conditions for sleep-disordered breathing

Obesity

Down syndrome

Craniofacial syndromes
- Craniosynostoses (Apert, Crouzon, Pfeiffer, and Saethre-Chotzen syndromes)
- Pierre Robin sequence
- Stickler syndrome
- CHARGE syndrome
- Mandibulofacial dysostotic (Treacher Collins syndrome)
- Craniofacial microsomia (hemifacial microsomia, Goldenhar syndrome, first and second branchial arch syndrome)
- Hallermann-Streiff syndrome

Mucopolysaccaridoses

Achondroplasia

Neuromuscular disease

Cerebral palsy

Beckwith-Weidemann syndrome

Klippel-Feil syndrome

Prader-Willi syndrome

Arnold-Chiari malformation

Sickle cell disease

Post pharyngoplasty patients

From Goldstein NA. Evaluation and management of pediatric obstructive sleep apnea. In: Flint PW, Lesperance MM, editors. Cumming pediatric otolaryngology. Philadelphia: Elsevier; 2015. p. 45–54; with permission.

Of these, PSG is considered the gold standard: the most reliable and objective measure of both the presence and severity of OSA. Parameters and ranges of normal for PSG are shown in **Box 2**. The most common parameter to ascertain OSA severity is the AHI, with most specialists considering this abnormal in children with an AHI greater than 1. An AHI greater than 5 is often considered as warranting tonsillectomy, but

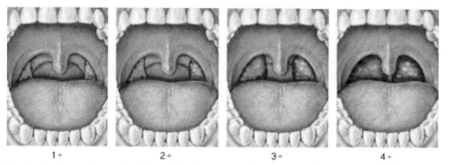

1+	2+	3+	4+

Fig. 2. Tonsil grading scale. (*From* Ball J, Daines JE, Flynn JA, et al. Ear, nose, and throat. In: Ball J, editor. Seidel's guide to physical examination. Philadelphia: Mosby; 2015. p. 231–59; with permission.)

Table 2
Gradation of tonsillar enlargement

Grade	Definition	Description
0	Not visible	Tonsils do not reach tonsillar pillars
1+	<25%	Tonsils fill <25% of the transverse oropharyngeal space measured between the anterior tonsillar pillars
2+	25% to 49%	Tonsils fill <50% of the transverse oropharyngeal space
3+	50% to 74%	Tonsils fill <75% of the transverse oropharyngeal space
4+	75% or more	Tonsils fill 75% or more of the transverse oropharyngeal space

From Baugh RF, Archer SM, Mitchell RB, et al. Clinical practice guideline: tonsillectomy in children. Otolaryngol Head Neck Surg 2011;144:S1–30; with permission.

Baugh and colleagues[1] note that there is not good evidence to base a cutoff value to indicate the need for tonsillectomy in children. Some children with AHI less than 5, with symptoms of SDB, may also meet indications for surgical intervention. Oxygen desaturation has also been shown to independently correlate with severity of OSA, specifically with a negative effect on academic performance.[1]

Clinical Decision Making - Clinical Practice Guidelines

The AAP, the AAO-HNS, and the Academy of Sleep Medicine have each recommended use of PSG in the evaluation of SDB, with the 2011 CPGs by the AAO-HNS the most specific guideline (**Table 3**). The AAO-HNS CPGs note that PSG can confirm the diagnosis of SDB as well as aid in perioperative planning by providing more specific knowledge regarding the severity of respiratory disruption. These CPGs can also assist in decision making when the need for surgery is uncertain, such as when there is discordance between physical examination findings and severity of caregiver-reported SDB symptoms, namely when tonsillar size is small but SDB symptoms are prominent or the reverse. In addition, the 2011 CPGs can be of use when there is difference of perspective between family members and clinicians regarding the relative need for surgery. Furthermore, the CPGs point out that in situations where "evidence is weak or benefits unclear" the patient preference in decision making should

Box 2
Abnormal values of pediatric polysomnography

Obstructive apnea index >1/h

AHI >1/h
  AHI 1 to 4 = mild
  AHI 5 to 10 = moderate
  AHI greater than 10 = severe

Peak end-tidal CO_2 greater than 53 mm Hg

End-tidal CO_2 greater than 50 mm Hg for more than 10% of total sleep time

Minimum oxyhemoglobin saturation below 92%

From Goldstein NA. Evaluation and management of pediatric obstructive sleep apnea. In: Flint PW, Lesperance MM, editors. Cumming pediatric otolaryngology. Philadelphia: Elsevier; 2015. p. 45–54; with permission.

Table 3
Summary action statement on polysomnography from 2011 American Academy of Otolaryngology–Head and Neck Surgery clinical practice guideline

Statement	Action	Evidence
1. Indications for PSG	Before performing tonsillectomy, the clinician should refer children with SDB for PSG if they exhibit any of the following: obesity. Down syndrome, craniofacial abnormalities, neuromuscular disorders, sickle cell disease, or mucopolysaccharidoses	Recommendation based on observational studies with a preponderance of benefit over harm
2. Advocating for PSG	The clinician should advocate for PSG prior to tonsillectomy for SDB in children without any of the comorbidities listed in statement 1 for whom the need for surgery is uncertain or when there is discordance between tonsillar size on physical examination and the reported severity of SDB.	Recommendation based on observational and case- control studies with a preponderance of benefit over harm
3. Communication with anesthesiologist	Clinicians should communicate PSG results to the anesthesiologist prior to the induction of anesthesia for tonsillectomy in a child with SDB.	Recommendation based on observational studies with a preponderance of benefit over harm
4. Inpatient admission for children with OSA documented in results of PSG	Clinicians should admit children with OSA documented in results of PSG for inpatient overnight monitoring after tonsillectomy If they are younger than age 3 or have severe OSA (AHI of 10 or more obstructive events/h. Oxygen saturation nadir <80% or both).	Recommendation based on observational studies with preponderance of benefit over harm
5. Unattended PSG with PM device	In children for whom PSG is indicated to assess SDB prior to tonsillectomy, clinicians should obtain laboratory-based PSG, when available.	Recommendation based on diagnostic studies with limitations and a preponderance of benefit over harm

From Baugh RF, Archer SM, Mitchell RB, et al. Clinical practice guideline: tonsillectomy in children. Otolaryngol Head Neck Surg 2011;144:S1–30; with permission.

be maximized and collaboration between the provider and the informed patient becomes even more important.[3]

Despite being the gold standard for diagnosis, PSG is not commonly ordered even among specialists, with an overwhelming majority of providers still basing need for surgery on their clinical evaluation.[34] Reasons for not ordering PSG may include PSG perceived as not reflecting the effects of SDB on a child's well-being, insufficient access to PSG testing and/or to pediatric PSG specialists (ie, child-friendly sleep laboratories), unwarranted cost, prolonging time to definitive treatment, and concern over the potential emotional distress of a child in the sleep laboratory.[1,3]

Specifically regarding PSG cost, Konka and colleagues[35] did an original study comparing the Clinical Assessment Score–15 instrument (CAS-15), a diagnostic tool that combines 10 history items and 5 physical examination items to calculate a score to aid in determining clinical indication for surgery, to PSG in diagnosis. That study found that that the CAS-15 was superior in cost-benefit even when compared in light of subsequent reduction of AHI, improvement in disease-specific measure of QOL, and improvement in standardized measure of behavior.[35]

As discussed previously, questionnaires have been developed to aid practitioners in diagnosis and determining the need for surgery. Their diagnostic value is limited, however, due to poor ability to differentiate between those with SDB and those without compared with PSG. This may be due to parents' difficulty in being aware of these symptoms in their children while the parents are sleeping. These surveys seem to have more value in showing impact of treatment on QOL after surgery.[28,30,31] Notwithstanding these limitations, questionnaires as a diagnostic aid may become a more used tool as indicated in a more recent study of the CAS-15 instrument.

Audio/video taping, overnight pulse oximetry, and portable monitoring (PM) have shown some benefit in determining need for surgery but to a much lesser extent than PSG. Recently, PM in particular has received increased attention.[3] PM, or home sleep apnea testing, however, has not yet received unbiased endorsement due to a diversity of invalidated devices on the market, few of which have been tested in children.[3,30,36] Also, PM devices are seen as inappropriate for measurement of SBD in high-risk children because they have primarily only been tested in otherwise healthy children.[3]

Treatments of Sleep-Disordered Breathing

Tonsillectomy

AT is recommended as first-line treatment of children with OSA and has been shown to improve many of the sequelae of SDB. These include improvement of behavioral and neurocognitive problems, school performance, QOL, enuresis, and growth failure[1,6,11,31] Adenoidectomy alone is not regarded as sufficient: the combination of both procedures has been shown to give superior results than either procedure in isolation.[31,37] A recent meta-analysis of AT by Chinnadurai and colleagues[6] compared AT to watchful waiting and confirmed the efficacy of AT but with noted reliance on short-term data (<12 months). In their 2011 guidelines, the AAO-HNS also point out that the sequelae improved by AT are usually multifactorial and therefore AT may only result in partial improvement, requiring further management postoperatively.[1]

The role and frequency of AT have fluctuated greatly over the past century. Whereas tonsillectomy was the most frequently performed surgery in the United States from 1915 to the 1960s, the AAO-HNS has noted that there was a decrease of approximately 50% from 1977 to 1989. With the primary indication for tonsillectomy evolving from recurrent tonsillitis to SBD, the rates have increased again since the 1980s. Currently more than 530,000 tonsillectomies are performed annually in children younger than 15 years old in the United States.[1] Tonsillectomy is currently a common procedure, accounting for more than 15% of all surgeries performed in children under the age of 15 years.[6] The current tonsillectomy rate is 0.53 per thousand children, with 1.46 per thousand children for combined tonsillectomy and adenoidectomy.[38] It was found in 2012 that tonsillectomy was the fourth most common procedure performed in the operating room among US hospitals for children ages 1 to 17 year old.[39]

Surgical techniques for adenotonsillectomy The most common AT surgical technique involves a total, or extracapsular, approach, meaning that the tonsils are completely removed from their surrounding fascia.[40] Historically, this was accomplished via a combination of sharp and blunt dissection. Currently, *Cummings Pediatric Otolaryngology* notes the most popular method is dissection of tonsillar tissue using monopolar electrocautery, which is believed to provide better hemostasis. Other newer modalities gaining some popularity include bipolar cautery, plasma excision (coblation), and the harmonic scalpel.[5] Although tonsillectomy (**Fig. 3**), is generally considered a straightforward procedure, complications are possible, with a primary perioperative risk of bleeding.[41,42] High-risk children require overnight admission/observation, including children under the age of 3, with severe OSA (AHI >10), and/or with other cardiopulmonary comorbidities.[5] Data regarding the safety of AT in children less than 2 years of age are limited and debate exists on the role of AT versus other modalities in this age group.[43]

Subtotal tonsillectomy, also known as *tonsillotomy*, as an alternative to total tonsillectomy, has gained popularity, with some evidence suggesting easier recovery and fewer postoperative complications. Studies indicating lower risk with tonsillotomy, however, seem limited by confounders in data collection related to study populations and variabilities in surgical techniques used. There is also some reticence to adopt this approach due to the risk of tonsillar regrowth after subtotal resection, opening the possibility for need for a revision or secondary procedure.[40,44,45]

Other treatment modalities CPAP has a role in the treatment of SDB in children with excessive risk for AT, who have residual OSA after AT, or who do not have significantly enlarged tonsils or adenoids. This modality uses patient-specific calibrated air pressure, delivered via a mask, to splint open the airway during sleep and is effective. Compared with the 1-time surgical procedure and limited recovery period involved in surgical therapy with AT, however, CPAP requires continuous nightly use, and poor compliance has been noted in young children and those with behavioral problems.[30,31] Weight control, oral appliances, night-time oxygen therapy, and treatment of any accompanying rhinitis are other medical therapy options, whereas maxillary advancement surgery and tracheostomy are less commonly used surgical treatments reserved for patients with craniofacial anomalies, persistent OSA after AT, and/or when AT is deemed inappropriate.[30,31,43]

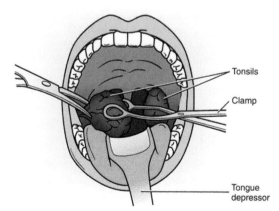

Fig. 3. Tonsillectomy. (*From* Otorhinolaryngologic and head and neck surgery. In: Phillips N, editor. Berry & Kohn's operating room technique. 11th edition. Philadelphia: Elsevier; 2007.)

SUMMARY

Despite general familiarity with tonsillectomy among medical providers, there is evidence that the specific indications and benefits of this surgery are not well known. SDB, the primary indication for tonsillectomy, has also been shown to be underestimated as a significant determining factor in the health of many children.[46–48] Future directions for research include obtaining an improved understanding of the incidence and impact of SDB on cardiovascular health, making PSG testing a more practical, better delineation of the ideal role for PSG in comparison to alternatives, such as PM and screening instruments, and performing a more fully controlled, comparative study of extracapsular (complete) tonsillectomy versus subtotal resection (tonsillotomy). Updates to current CPGs are anticipated to be released in spring of 2018 by the AAO-HNS, which may provide further clarity for providers who care for children with SDB.

ACKNOWLEDGMENTS

Dr. Jacob G. Robison, Pediatric Otolaryngologist at St. Luke's Children's Hospital in Boise Idaho, provided valuable feedback and direction on this article. His professional insight and encouragement was greatly appreciated.

REFERENCES

1. Baugh RF, Archer SM, Mitchell RB, et al. Clinical practice guideline: tonsillectomy in children. Otolaryngol Head Neck Surg 2011;144:S1–30.
2. Tonsillectomy facts in the U.S.: from ENT doctors. 2009. Available at: http://www.entnet.org/content/tonsillectomy-facts-us-ent-doctors. Accessed June 11, 2017.
3. Roland PS, Rosenfeld RM, Brooks LJ. Clinical practice guideline: polysomnography for sleep-disordered breathing prior to tonsillectomy in children. Otolaryngol Head Neck Surg 2011;145:S1–15.
4. Lumeng JC, Chervin RD. Epidemiology of pediatric obstructive sleep apnea. Proc Am Thorac Soc 2008;5:242–52.
5. Goldstein NA. Evaluation and management of pediatric obstructive sleep apnea. In: Flint PW, Lesperance MM, editors. Cummings pediatric otolaryngology. Philadelphia: Elsevier; 2015. p. 45–54.
6. Chinnadurai S, Jordan AK, Sathe NA, et al. Tonsillectomy for obstructive sleep disordered breathing: a meta-analysis. Pediatrics 2017;139(2) [pii:e20163491].
7. Beebe DW. Neurobehavioral morbidity associated with disordered breathing during sleep in children: a comprehensive review. Sleep 2006;29:1115–34.
8. Gruber R, Xi T, Frenette S, et al. Sleep disturbances in prepubertal children with attention deficit hyperactivity disorder: a home polysomnography study. Sleep 2009;32(3):343–50.
9. Constantin E, Low NCP, Dugas E, et al. Association between childhood sleep-disordered breathing and disruptive behavior disorders in childhood and adolescence. Behav Sleep Med 2015;13(6):442–54.
10. Owens JA. Neurocognitive and behavioral impact of sleep disordered breathing in children. Pediatr Pulmonol 2009;44(5):417–22.
11. Marcus CL, Moore RH, Rosen CL, et al. A randomized trial of adenotonsillectomy for childhood sleep apnea. N Engl J Med 2013;368(25):2366–76.
12. Gozal D. Sleep-disordered breathing and school performance in children. Pediatrics 1998;102:612–20.

13. Galland B, Spruyt K, Dawes P, et al. Sleep disordered breathing and academic performance: a meta-analysis. Pediatrics 2015;136:e935–46.
14. Graham K, Levy J. Enuresis. Pediatr Rev 2009;30(5):165–72.
15. Jeyakumar A, rahman S, Armbrecht E, et al. The association between sleep-disordered breathing and enuresis in children. Laryngoscope 2012;122: 1873–7.
16. Wang RC, Elkins TP, Keech D, et al. Accuracy of clinical evaluation in pediatric obstructive sleep apnea. Otolaryngol Head Neck Surg 1998;118:69–73.
17. Williams E, Woo P, Miller R, et al. The effects of adenotonsillectomy on growth in young children. Otolaryngol Head Neck Surg 1991;104:509–16.
18. Cole SZ, Lanham JS. Failure to thrive: an update. Am Fam Physician 2011;83: 829–34.
19. Bonuck K, Parikh S, Bassila M, et al. Growth failure and sleep disordered breathing: a review of the literature. Int J Pediatr Otorhinolaryngol 2006;70:769–78.
20. Smith DF, Vikani AR, Benke JR, et al. Weight gain after adenotonsillectomy is more common in young children. Otolaryngol Head Neck Surg 2013;148:488–93.
21. Bonuck KA, Freeman K, Henderson J. Growth and growth biomarker changes after adenotonsillectomy: systematic review and meta-analysis. Arch Dis Child 2009;94:83–91.
22. Jeyakumar A, Fettman N, Armbrecht E, et al. A systematic review of adenotonsillectomy as a risk factor for childhood obesity. Otolaryngol Head Neck Surg 2011; 144:154–8.
23. Paul GR, Pinto S. Sleep and the cardiovascular system in children. Sleep Med Clin 2017;12:179–91.
24. Teo DT, Mitchell RB. Systematic review of effects of adenotonsillecotmy on cardiovascular parameters in children with obstructive sleep apnea. Otolaryngol Head Neck Surg 2013;148:21–8.
25. Nisbet LC, Yiallaruorou SR, Walter LM, et al. Blood pressure regulation, autonomic control and sleep disordered breathing in children. Sleep Med Rev 2014;18:179–89.
26. Ehsan Z, Ishman S, Kimball TR, et al. Longitudinal cardiovascular outcomes of sleep disordered breathing in children: a meta-analysis and systematic review. Sleep 2017;40(3).
27. Vlahandonis A, Walter LM, Horne RSC. Does treatment of SDB in children improve cardiovascular outcome? Sleep Med Rev 2013;17:75–85.
28. Garetz SL. Behavior, cognition, and quality of life after adenotonsillectomy for pediatric sleep-disordered breathing: summary of the literature. Otolaryngol Head Neck Surg 2008;138:S19–26.
29. Franco RA, Roenfeld RM, Madu R. Quality of life for children with obstructive sleep apnea. Otolaryngol Head Neck Surg 2000;123:9–16.
30. Sinha D, Guilleminault C. Sleep disordered breathing in children. Indian J Med Res 2010;131:311–20.
31. Section on Pediatric Pulmonology, Subcommittee on Obstructive Sleep Apnea Syndrome. American Academy of Pediatrics. Clinical pratice guidlines: diagnosis and management of childhood obstructive sleep apnea syndrome. Pediatrics 2002;109:704–12.
32. Nation J, Brigger M. The efficacy of adenotonsillectomy for obstructive sleep apnea in children with Down syndrome: a systematic review. Otolaryngol Head Neck Surg 2017;157:1–8.
33. Guilleminault C, Lee HJ, Chan A. Pediatric obstructive sleep apnea syndrome. Arch Pediatr Adolesc Med 2005;159:775–85.

34. Friedman NR, Perkins JN, McNair MS, et al. Current practice patterns for sleep-disordered breathing in children. Laryngoscope 2013;123:1055–9.

35. Konka A, Weedon J, Goldstein NA. Cost-benefit analysis of polysomnography versus clinical assessment score-15 (CAS-15) for treatment of pediatric sleep-disordered breathing. Otolaryngol Head Neck Surg 2014;151:484–8.

36. Tan HL, Kheirandish-Gozal L, Gozal D. Pediatric home sleep apnea testing: slowing getting there! Chest 2015;148:1382–95.

37. Guilleminault C, Li KK, Kharamtosov A, et al. Sleep disordered breathing: surgical outcomes in prepubertal children. Laryngoscope 2004;114:132–7.

38. Bhattacharyya N, Lin HW. Changes and consistencies in the epidemiology of pediatric adenotonsillar surgery, 1996-2006. Otolaryngol Head Neck Surg 2010; 143:680–4.

39. Fingar KR, Stocks C, Weiss AJ, et al. Most frequent operating room procedures performed in U.S. Hospitals, 2003-2012. Rockville (MD): Healthcare Cost and Utilization Project; 2014. Available at: https://www.hcup-us.ahrq.gov/reports/statbriefs/sb186-Operating-Room-Procedures-United-States-2012.jsp.

40. Sathe N, Chinnadurai S, McPheeters M, et al. Comparative effectiveness of partial versus total tonsillectomy in children: a systematic review. Otolaryngol Head Neck Surg 2017;156(3):456–63.

41. Francis DO, Fonnesbeck C, Sathe N, et al. Postoperative bleeding and associated utilization following tonsillectomy in children: a systematic review and meta-analysis. Otolaryngol Head Neck Surg 2017;156(3):442–55.

42. Mattos JL, Robison JG, Greenberg J, et al. Acetaminophen plus ibuprofen versus opioids for treatment of post-tonsillectomy pain in children. Int J Pediatr Otorhinolaryngol 2014;78:1671–6.

43. Robison JG, Wilson C, Otteson TD, et al. Analysis of outcomes in treatment of obstructive sleep apnea in infants. Laryngoscope 2013;123:2306–14.

44. Windfur JP, Savva K, Dahm JD, et al. Tonsillotomy: facts and fiction. Eur Arch Otorhinolaryngol 2015;272:949–69.

45. Wood JM, Cho M, Carney AS. Role of subtotal tonsillectomy ('tonsillotomy') in children with sleep disordered breathing. J Laryngol Otol 2014;128:S3–7.

46. Bauer EE, Lee R, Campbell YN. Preoperative screening for sleep-disordered breathing in children: a systematic literature review. AORN J 2016;104:542–50.

47. Gundnadottir G, Ehnhage A, Bende M, et al. Healthcare provider contact for children with symptoms of sleep-disordered breathing: a population survery. J Laryngol Otol 2016;130:296–301.

48. Kilaikode S, Weiss M, Megalaa R, et al. Distinguishing characteristics of severe obstructive sleep apnea in inner-city children and adolescents. Am J Respir Crit Care Med 2017;195.

Pediatric Otitis Media
An Update

Laura A. Kirk, MSPAS, PA-C

KEYWORDS

- Acute otitis media • Clinical practice guidelines • Eustachian tube dysfunction
- Middle ear effusion • Myringotomy • Pediatric hearing loss • Pediatric otitis media
- Otitis media with effusion

KEY POINTS

- Nearly all preschool age children are impacted by acute otitis media or otitis media with effusion.
- Treatment goals in the management of acute otitis media must be weighed against the side effects of antibiotics.
- There is an opportunity for reeducation and redirection of clinicians toward evidence-based medicine in this most common of conditions.

INTRODUCTION

Otitis medias are common, affecting most children, with more than 2 million episodes of middle ear fluid diagnosed per year in the United States. This diagnosis is second only to upper respiratory infection as the most common illness for which children receive a professional diagnosis.[1,2] However, after a clinical practice guideline (CPG) on acute otitis media was jointly released in 2004 with great fanfare and publicity by the American Academy of Pediatrics (AAP) and American Academy of Family Practice (AAFP), no significant changes in practice patterns were noted when comparing surveys of primary care providers in 2002 with those in 2006, indicating that clinicians are either unaware of or hesitant to follow the guidelines.[2] Also, in 2013, only some pediatricians were found to follow otitis media with effusion CPGs, released in 2004 by the American Academy of Otolaryngology–Head and Neck Surgery (AAO-HNS) in collaboration with AAP and AAFP.[3,4] There is clearly an opportunity for reeducation and redirection of clinicians toward evidence-based medicine in this common condition.

I have no commercial or financial conflicts of interest nor any funding sources relevant to this article's content.
Department of Otolaryngology–Head and Neck Surgery, UCSF Medical Center, 2380 Sutter Street, San Francisco, CA 94115, USA
E-mail address: Laura.Kirk@UCSF.edu

Physician Assist Clin 3 (2018) 207–222
https://doi.org/10.1016/j.cpha.2017.11.004

TERMINOLOGY

Normal middle ears are a mucosal membrane–lined cavity filled with air, allowing free vibration of both tympanic membrane (TM) and the ossicular chain of middle ear bones, which pass vibratory sound to the cochlea (**Fig. 1**). Otitis media, or inflammation of the middle ear, is so common that it has been called an "occupational hazard of early childhood,"[5] with an average of 4 episodes per year,[6] with only 10% of children entering kindergarten never having had middle ear fluid.[7] When this middle ear fluid becomes secondarily infected with resulting inflammation of the middle ear (ME) and TM, the condition is called *acute otitis media* (AOM), colloquially known as an *ear infection* (**Fig. 2**). However, serous fluid can also remain in the middle ear without signs or symptoms of infection, which is known as *otitis media with effusion* (OME), or simply *ear fluid* (**Fig. 3**).

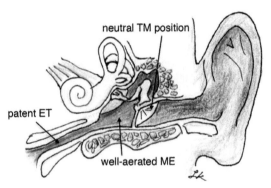

Fig. 1. A well-aerated middle ear cavity facilitates transmission of sound vibration most efficiently from external ear, through the tympanic membrane, then the ossicular chain, and into the cochlea.

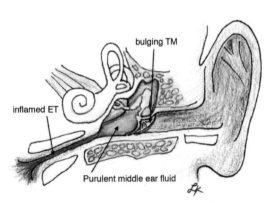

Fig. 2. Middle ear inflammation with secondary infection of ME fluid is called *acute otitis media*. The tympanic membrane bulges outward because of increased ME pressure.

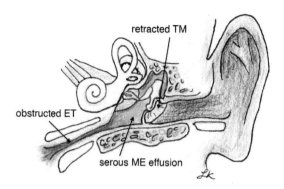

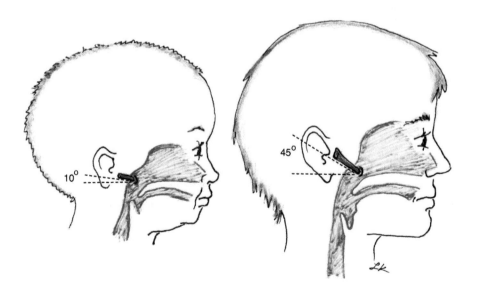

Fig. 3. Persistent fluid in the middle ear cavity and negative pressure caused by nonfunctioning Eustachian tube creates retraction and immobility of the TM.

ANATOMY OF A CHILDHOOD EPIDEMIC

It is the geometry of a child's Eustachian tube (ET) that is largely to blame for otitis media: this dynamic ventilating structure is oriented horizontally in infancy, with a gradually more vertical orientation during childhood as the jaw and neck progressively elongate. This elongation results in increased tone and length of the ET to better aerate and protect the middle ear (**Fig. 4**).

RISK FACTORS

Any inflammation of the mucosal membranes of the nasopharynx, such as in a respiratory infection, seasonal allergic reactivity, or laryngopharyngeal reflux, may lead to

Fig. 4. The Eustachian tube of an infant is unfavorable for middle ear health, as it is shorter, floppier, and nearly horizontal at 10°, compared with that of an adult, which is longer, more firm, and angled (45°).

swelling of the mucosal ET lining and partial or complete occlusion of the tube lumen. This condition leads to accumulation of natural secretions of the middle ear mucosa and the buildup of negative pressure, which further draws fluid into the middle ear space. Risk factors for ET dysfunction from inflammation also include time spent in day care with greater than 3 children, frequent colds, second-hand tobacco smoke exposure, laryngopharyngeal reflux, and early introduction of cow's milk.[8,9] Anatomic variations that are unfavorable for ET function thereby increasing risk of middle ear fluid, include enlarged adenoids, which obstruct the ET orifice; syndromes with cranio-facial anomalies, which shorten the nasopharynx; and cleft palate, which limits natural movements of the musculature surrounding the ET orifice (**Table 1**).

EPIDEMIOLOGY OF OTITIS MEDIA

The natural history for middle ear fluid in a child is one of gradual spontaneous res-olution within 3 months, with a mean duration of 17 days per episode.[6] However, fluid can recur episodically in 30% to 40% of children or even persist for more than a year in 5% to 10% of children.[7,10,11] Children are most prone to middle ear effusion (MEE) from birth to age 2 years with 60% incidence, which decreases to 1 in 8 children age 5 to 6 years.[12,13] At least a quarter of ME fluid persists for more than 3 months.[14]

IMPACT AT HOME

Serous middle ear fluid is often undetected in early childhood but is not necessarily asymptomatic; the resultant decreased mobility of the tympanic membrane and reduced vibratory transmission of sound through a fluid-encased ossicular chain lead to conductive hearing loss and increasing risk of delayed speech and language acquisition. Middle ear fluid can also cause vestibular balance disruption, which may present as delayed ambulation or increased falls. Parents of children with OME prospectively surveyed reported that 76% experienced otalgia, 64% had sleep disruption, 49% had behavioral challenges, between one-third and two-thirds had speech and hearing concerns, and 15% struggled with imbalance.[15] OME also in-creases the risk of AOM with up to 5 times higher rate of ear infection when a baseline effusion is present.[16] Caregivers of children with OME report high levels of worry and inconvenience, and parent-child interactions may be poorer.[15–17]

OTOLOGIC IMPACT

Pediatric hearing impairment in developed nations is most commonly caused by OME, although permanent hearing loss from otitis media is rare.[18,19] Middle ear effusions contain inflammatory mediators, which cause local, reactive changes in the TM and

Table 1 Risk factors for Eustachian tube dysfunction and otitis media with effusion	
Anatomic Factors	**Environmental/Exposure Factors**
Cleft palate	Allergic rhinitis
Craniofacial syndromes	Upper respiratory tract illness
Male gender	with/without AOM
Genetic predisposition	Second-hand smoke exposure
	Day care
	Not breastfeeding
	No pneumococcal vaccination

middle ear. Sequelae of Eustachian tube dysfunction (ETD), untreated OME, and recurrent AOMs include TM perforation, progressive retraction of the TM, retraction pockets of the TM, adherence of TM to the ossicles, ossicular erosion, and formation of cholesteatoma skin cysts, which risks more profound erosive changes of the middle and even inner ear. Rarely, serious and potentially life-threatening complications can occur from untreated AOM, including mastoiditis, meningitis, and intracranial abscesses.

HEALTH CARE BURDEN

The health care burden of OME and AOM is significant: 2.2 million new cases of OME are diagnosed annually in the United States and otitis medias (OME and AOM) account for 1 in 9 primary care office visits.[5,20] The direct costs of care for otitis medias are between $3 billion and $5 billion annually. Indirect costs are large but difficult to estimate, particularly decreased caregiver productivity.[16,21–23] Medical therapies attempting to alleviate middle ear fluid are largely ineffective, as discussed later in this article, but these treatment efforts increase the direct costs of managing otitis media. As mentioned in this article's introduction, although otitis media is common, surveillance studies of pediatric practices indicate that few clinicians actually follow established clinical practice guidelines, particularly for children with OME, potentially increasing costs of care unnecessarily.[3,4]

CLINICAL PRACTICE GUIDELINES TO GUIDE EVIDENCE-BASED CARE

The remainder of this article discusses clinical practice guidelines related to AOM and OME and indications for tympanostomy tube placement, with particular attention to the most frequently misunderstood guideline recommendations. The strength of action terms in guidelines varies based on the quality of available evidence: strong recommendation (A), recommendation (B), option (O), no recommendation (N), or recommendation against (X) (**Table 2**).

DIFFERENTIATION BETWEEN OTITIS MEDIAS: OTOSCOPY

Otitis media with effusion may result from or contribute to development of acute otitis media. The 2 types of otitis media are on a continuum.[24]

Assessing the position of the dynamic tympanic membrane in relationship to the static bony landmarks of the middle ear is of utmost importance in diagnosing and differentiating between otitis medias. A normal tympanic membrane rests neutrally draped over the stable framework of the annulus and malleus (**Fig. 5**). Compare this with the retracted appearance of a tympanic membrane in the setting of inadequate

Table 2 Strength in action terms in guidelines		
	Recommendation	Evidence Quality and Risk vs Benefit
A	Strong recommendation	High-quality evidence shows clear benefit
B	Recommendation	Good-quality evidence shows benefit > harm
O	Option	Balance of benefit and harm, and/or weaker evidence
N	No recommendation	Weak or insufficient evidence for guidance
X	Recommendation against	Evidence clearly unfavorable for this action

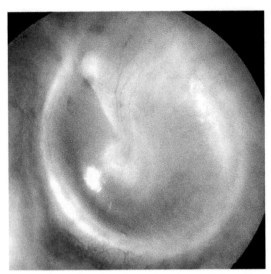

Fig. 5. A normal TM rests neutrally draped over the circumference of the medial ear canal and the malleus.

Eustachian tube ventilation, which becomes concave, pulled into the middle ear cavity (**Fig. 6**). In most cases of AOM, the TM bulges outward in relationship to bony landmarks, is convex in appearance, and is pushed toward the viewer by a building volume of purulence in the middle ear cavity (**Fig. 7**).

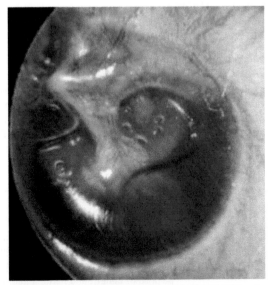

Fig. 6. In a middle ear with poor ventilation by the Eustachian tube, retraction can develop, pulling the TM deep into the middle ear and making bony landmarks appear more prominent. Often golden, serous ME fluid forms, with air-fluid levels seen in this image.

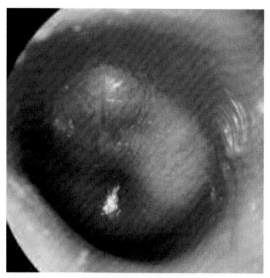

Fig. 7. As pressure from infected middle ear fluid builds, the TM is pushed outward in acute otitis media, obscuring natural bony landmarks. Often the TM is erythematous, and sometimes the ME fluid can be seen to be purulent, as in this image.

DIFFERENTIATION BETWEEN OTITIS MEDIAS: PNEUMATIC OTOSCOPY

In both AOM and OME, middle ear effusion is present and should be confirmed based on pneumatic otoscopy or tympanometry (A-B) to confirm lack of visible or measurable TM movement.[25,26] All children who have otalgia, hearing loss, or both should be evaluated with pneumatic otoscopy (A).[26] Any clinician routinely evaluating children in a primary care context, including urgent or emergent care settings, should therefore have a pneumatic bulb attachment to their otoscope to facilitate this examination. The examiner's hand that holds the otoscope speculum must be braced against the child's head, then a speculum slightly wider than the ear canal is inserted and angled to achieve an air-tight seal in the outer (cartilaginous) ear canal. Gently squeezing and releasing the bulb to create positive and negative air pressure against the TM allows dynamic assessment of the aeration of the middle ear. If there is an MEE, the positive and negative pressure application causes merely wrinkling or barely perceptible TM movements or can bring an air-fluid level into clearer visibility.

BARRIERS TO EVALUATION

Even practiced efforts at a thorough examination of a child's tympanic membrane can have numerous pitfalls, including lack of necessary equipment such as a well-lit otoscope with pneumatic bulb and appropriate-sized speculae attachments to facilitate a snug seal with the lateral ear canal. The young pediatric patient is often resistant to examination, skilled assistance in restraining the child may not be available, and the ear(s) may have cerumen within the canal, which obstructs full visualization of the TM. When these barriers cannot be eliminated, guidelines acknowledge that diagnosis must be based on patient context and individualized decision making.[25,26]

OTITIS MEDIA WITH EFFUSION
Diagnosis of Otitis Media with Effusion

Chronic OME is diagnosed when a child has middle ear fluid present for 3 or more months, based on either caregiver-reported onset of symptoms or diagnostic examination of ME fluid without infection. Pneumatic otoscopy is strongly recommended to determine presence of fluid, but when results of this clinical examination are uncertain because of technique, equipment, incomplete visualization because of cerumen or a narrow canal or if the child does not tolerate the examination, then tympanometry should be obtained for improved diagnostic accuracy (A).[26]

All newborns in the United States are screened for hearing loss before leaving the hospital postpartum. Of those infants who failed hearing screening (which prompts a referral for further testing), 55% had OME.[27] Middle ear fluid in infancy is typically a transient finding, but it does not rule out an underlying, unrelated sensorineural hearing loss, so repeat examination and hearing testing is warranted to confirm the etiology (or etiologies) of the hearing loss.

Otitis Media with Effusion in At-risk Children

Children with sensory, physical, or behavioral deficits are already at risk for speech, language, or learning delays. At-risk children should be screened for ME fluid at diagnosis of deficit and again at 12 and 18 months of age, as this is a critical developmental period (B)[26] (**Table 3**). When at-risk children have an MEE, they are disproportionally impacted by the added sensory comorbidity, so a hearing test should be performed. Placement of tympanostomy tubes should be offered if the likelihood of spontaneous resolution of fluid is thought to be low.[28] If no intervention is pursued, the child should be monitored frequently, with evaluation at least every 3 months. Outside of routine ear examinations during well-child visits, children who are not at risk and who are asymptomatic do not need special screening for OME (B).

Observation of Otitis Media with Effusion

Once ME fluid is noted on examination, the child who is not at risk should be examined again 3 months from date of onset of symptoms (if known) or 3 months from diagnosis (A). As ME fluid is often self-limited, particularly if present because of common environmental or temporary exposure to risk factors, watchful waiting in 3-month intervals helps avoid unnecessary intervention.[1,26] If fluid persists beyond 3 months, then age-appropriate hearing testing is warranted. Observation every 3 to 6 months should continue until the fluid resolves, significant hearing loss develops, or degree of TM or ME abnormalities from chronic OME become concerning (B).[26] During this time, parents and teachers should be counseled as to the potential impact ME fluid can have on speech, language, and learning (B).[26] Families should be made aware of suggested accommodations: optimal listening environments by preferential seating of child close to the teacher in class, speaking clearly and directly to the child, limiting background noise, and repeating verbal communications as needed for

Table 3		
At-risk children		
Sensory	**Physical**	**Behavioral**
Permanent hearing loss	Cleft palate	Autism spectrum
Visual impairment	Genetic syndrome	Pervasive developmental delay
Speech/language delay	Craniofacial anomaly	

misunderstandings. In children who are not at risk and who have minimal hearing loss or who have had no obvious impact on quality of life from OME, shared decision making with caregivers is of utmost importance, and observation of the MEE may be elected indefinitely.

Medical Therapy for Otitis Media with Effusion

There is limited, if any, role for medical therapy in management of OME. Intranasal steroids, systemic steroids, antibiotics, antihistamines, or decongestants should not be used to treat OME based on high-quality studies (X). Unless there is a coexisting condition (such as allergic rhinitis, in which case intranasal steroid spray and antihistamines could be appropriate), these medical therapies have no proven benefit for resolving ME fluid or improving hearing loss from OME.[29] Each medical therapy incurs unnecessary cost and side effects for the treatment of a usually self-limited condition.

Further Interventions for Otitis Media with Effusion

Middle ear effusions are less likely to spontaneously resolve if the date of onset is unknown or more than 6 months prior, the onset of OME was during summer or fall, the worse ear's hearing loss is ≥30 dB, a child has a history of prior tympanostomy tubes, and/or there has been no prior adenoidectomy.[30] Children may not be able to effectively autoinflate the Eustachian tube and middle ear with a Valsalva maneuver, but Politzer medical devices such as OtoVent (Abigo Medical, Askim, Sweden) or EarPopper (Summit Medical, St Paul, Minnesota, USA) are safe, may make ET and ME self-ventilation easier, and have modest short-term data supporting their use.

Tympanostomy Tubes

If the middle ear is not adequately ventilated spontaneously or via the above conservative interventions, then surgical measures may be considered. In the youngest patients, recent data regarding risks of general anesthesia for children less than 3 years of age must be weighed with the impact OME has on each particular patient. Placement of tympanostomy tubes, also known as *pressure equalization* (PE) *tubes, ventilation tubes*, or simply *ear tubes* is the most common reason for children in the United States to undergo anesthesia.[31] The purpose of a PE tube is to maintain a patent myringotomy to provide sustained ventilation of the middle ear or facilitate delivery of topical otic therapies into the middle ear. Although the procedure is quick (10–15 minutes), minimally painful, and tolerated by most adults in an outpatient setting, pediatric patients require a brief anesthesia for myringotomy and tube placement. After a myringotomy incision is made through the anteroinferior TM, any existing fluid is suctioned free from the middle ear, then a tube is inserted (**Fig. 8**). The ear is then filled with otic drops to cleanse residual ME fluid and maintain tube patency. Tubes with small phlanges, commonly known as grommet or Reuter bobbin tubes, maintain tube position by phlanges resting on either side of the TM, for an average duration of 1 year in situ. The natural process of TM exfoliation and epithelial migration gradually extrudes the tube posterolaterally into the ear canal, closing the myringotomy beneath the extruding tube. Longer-lasting tubes with larger flanges such as T tubes can be used for patients with chronic ETD who are expected to need assistance in middle ear ventilation for longer periods.

Risks and Complications of Pressure Equalization Tubes

Clinical practice guidelines were developed by the AAO-HNS in 2013 on tympanostomy tubes in children to weigh risks versus benefits of tube placement in various clinical scenarios.[28] Placement of PE tubes is a common procedure, but not without cost

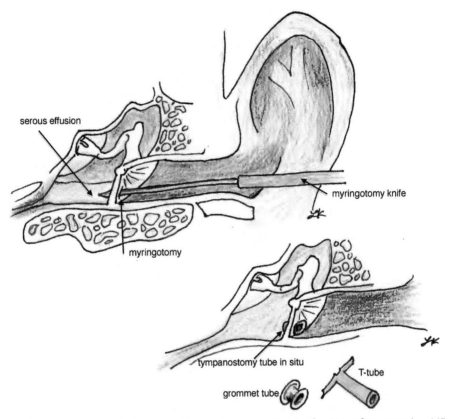

Fig. 8. A myringotomy knife is used to create an opening in the TM. After removing ME fluid, a tympanostomy tube is inserted into the myringotomy to maintain ventilation of the middle ear. Short-acting grommet tubes have small flanges on either side of the TM. Longer-acting T tubes have longer tube length and longer flanges, which sit on the medial side of the TM.

and risk. Average cost of the procedure is $2700 in the United States, which is cost effective for pediatric otitis media, based on a chart review in one managed care organization.[32] The most common complication of tympanostomy tubes is otorrhea, with 26% incidence.[33] Acute otorrhea in the setting of tubes is usually cleared easily with topical otic antibiotic therapy (such as ofloxacin otic drops), which provide much higher antibiotic concentration at the site of infection compared with systemic therapy. Therefore, acute otorrhea from patent tubes should not be treated with systemic antibiotics as part of initial therapy (X), but oral antibiotics can be considered in the case of prolonged otorrhea (>4 weeks), failure of topical otic therapy, or regional symptoms accompanying otorrhea.[28,34]

Other complications from PE tubes are rare, such as morbidity and mortality from anesthesia, or uncommon such as early extrusion of tube, tube occlusion, granulation tissue formation, prolonged retention of tube, persistent perforation of TM after tube extrusion, myringosclerosis (scarring of TM), medialization of tube into middle ear, or recurrence of OME after tube extrusion with need for replacement tube(s). To monitor children for complications from PE tubes, they should be evaluated 2 to 3 times per year, commonly via semiannual tube checks by otolaryngology provider.

Water exposure for children with PE tubes does not place them at higher risk for otorrhea, so avoidance of water sports or use of ear plugs is not necessary (X).[28]

Indications for Pressure Equalization Tubes in Otitis Media with Effusion

Tympanostomy tubes are beneficial for pediatric OME, as defined by MEE present for 3 months or more, when mild to moderate conductive hearing loss from the MEE is also present, as ventilation of the ME results in improvement in hearing in age-appropriate audiologic testing (A).[26,28] Per CPG for OME, if no hearing loss is present in a child with OME, then they should be observed in 3- to 6- month intervals until effusions resolve, hearing loss develops, or concerning changes in TM (namely significant retraction) occur because of chronic ETD (B). Tubes are not recommended if MEE has not been present for less than 3 months (X). It is an option to consider placement of tubes in children with MEE in one or both ears for more than 3 months who are symptomatic, with balance of benefit with harm and emphasis placed on shared decision making with caregivers (O).[28]

ACUTE OTITIS MEDIA
Diagnosis of Acute Otitis Media

One of the first, and most important steps in the clinical diagnosis of AOM is to distinguish AOM from OME. A child presenting with otalgia and an injected TM, in the absence of middle ear fluid (based on pneumatic otoscopy), does not have AOM. The diagnosis of AOM should be rendered when there is moderate to severe bulging of the TM (B). If there is only mild TM bulging, then there should be a history of recent (<48 hours) onset of otalgia or intense erythema of the TM present to diagnose AOM (B). Use of these more stringent otoscopic criteria is a change away from the 2004 guidelines' category of diagnostic uncertainty. The 2013 CPG on Diagnosis and Management of AOM emphasizes importance of otoscopy, discussing the lack of sensitivity of visual pain scales or symptom scores (such as ear tugging/manipulation, excessive crying, difficulty sleeping, irritability, decreased appetite, and fever) in accurately diagnosing AOM.[35,36] However, symptom scores have value in tracking clinical response to therapy over time, and an assessment of pain is very important (A).[25,37]

Management of the Pain of Acute Otitis Media

It is strongly recommended that the otalgia that is commonly present in AOM is noted and managed (A). Children younger than 2 years of age may have pain for a longer duration than older children.[38] Numerous studies show that antibiotic therapy alone does not rapidly (within 24 hours) reduce pain, so analgesics should be prescribed (with or without antibiotic therapy) and continued as long as necessary.[39] There is no preponderance of evidence for one oral analgesic over another in the treatment of AOM, so the 2004 and 2013 CPG leave this to the clinician's best judgment regarding risks and benefits, incorporating parent/patient preferences.[25]

Evidence of anesthetic topical otic therapy versus placebo (saline or homeopathic) ear drops suggests low likelihood of complications in an ear with intact TM, but inconsistent response or no statistically significant difference.[40,41] In 2015, 1 month after publication of an animal study on Auralgan (benzocaine and antipyrine over-the-counter ear drops) instilled into chinchilla's middle ears found ototoxic effects,[42] the US Food and Drug Administration (FDA) announced its "intention to take enforcement action against companies that manufacture and/or distribute certain unapproved prescription ear drop products (known as otic products) labeled to relieve ear pain, infection, and inflammation."[43]

Antibiotic Therapy for Acute Otitis Media

An exhaustive discussion of antibiotic therapy for AOM is beyond the scope of this article. Antibiotic therapy is warranted because of the high prevalence of bacteria found in the ME fluid of children at the time of AOM diagnosis based on tympanocentesis as well as a meta-analysis finding the absolute rates of clinical improvement with treatment.[44,45] For most patients, first-line therapy is high-dose amoxicillin, as it is narrow spectrum with good efficacy against common pathogens, safe, and inexpensive and has an inoffensive taste.[46] For children who have had amoxicillin within the 30 days before current AOM or those with concurrent conjunctivitis, high-dose amoxicillin-clavulanate is recommended for broader coverage (B).[25] For children who are penicillin allergic, cephalosporins are a reasonable choice, as cross-reactivity to cephalosporins has been found to be significantly lower than the historically reported 10%, particularly in the case of second- or third-generation cephalosporins, such as cefdinir and cefuroxime.[47] If parents report no improvement or worsening symptoms at 48 to 72 hours after antibiotic is initiated, the child should be reassessed (B). Treatment failures can be treated with these oral antibiotic alternatives to amoxicillin discussed above, or intramuscular cephalexin, with a 3-day course of cephalexin more effective than a single dose.[48] It is unclear what duration of therapy is optimal; the typical 10-day therapy regimen for AOM was extrapolated from treatment recommendations for streptococcal pharyngitis. The younger the child, the more favorable a 10-day treatment course, with a 5- to 7-day course likely adequate for children older than 6 years.[49]

The goals of antibiotic therapy are to expedite elimination of the acute middle ear infection, to prevent regional or systemic acute infectious complications (such as mastoiditis and meningitis), and to minimize risk of chronic local complications of AOM such as cholesteatoma. Treatment with antibiotics is found in most studies to decrease duration of otalgia, analgesic use, or school and work absence for patients and caregivers, respectively.[50,51] The 2013 CPG on AOM incorporates new studies with stringent diagnostic criteria and observational studies regarding natural history in untreated children. Based on these results, there is now a choice of either initial observation or initial antibiotic therapy in children ages 6 months to 2 years, even with certain diagnosis of unilateral AOM, as long as symptoms are not severe and caregivers are in agreement with this watch-and-wait plan (B).[25] This period of watchful waiting allows for confirmation that viral otitis media has indeed become secondarily infected with bacteria before initiating antibiotics, as viral AOMs tend to spontaneously resolve within 48 hours.

Management of Recurrent Acute Otitis Media

Recurrent AOM by definition is a frequency of at least 3 separate episodes of AOM in 6 months or 4 episodes in 1 year (including 1 in the preceding 6 months). There is NO role for prophylactic antibiotic therapy for recurrent episodes of AOM (B).[25] Risks of long-term antibiotic use outweigh the potential benefit, which was found to be a reduction but not elimination of infections, and there is also a high number needed to treat to prevent a single AOM.[52] Using prevention measures against AOM should be considered, such as pneumococcal and influenza vaccinations (A-B), exclusive breastfeeding for 6 months or more (B), and avoidance of tobacco smoke exposure (B).[25] There is insufficient evidence for recommendations against bottle propping, pacifier use, and attending child care, although each is associated with increased rates of AOMs (N).[25]

Indications for Tympanostomy Tubes in Acute Otitis Media

Consideration of surgical intervention is an option for a child with recurrent or persistent AOM, although it is more controversial than for the child with OME. Myringotomy with placement of tympanostomy tubes is the most common first-line surgical option. The efficacy of tubes to prevent recurrence of AOMs is not proven, as systematic reviews show insufficient evidence with small short-term benefit.[53,54] However, placement of PE tubes when there is not MEE present between infections is not recommended, as risk outweighs benefit (X).[28] Exceptions may be made in favor of tube placement without baseline OME in the case of children at high risk: those who are syndromic, who are developmentally delayed, with sensory (especially visual and underlying auditory) deficits, with learning disabilities, with immune deficiencies, and/or with multiple or severe antibiotic allergies (O).[26,28]

Therapy for Otitis Media: Future Directions for Research

Amoxicillin-clavulanate's broader spectrum of coverage may prove a preferable initial choice over high-dose amoxicillin if high-quality studies using today's more stringent diagnostic criteria can show greater efficacy.[25] Treatment goals in the management of AOM must be weighed against the side effects of antibiotics. Development of resistant strains of bacteria, as well as significant and prolonged alteration of the aerodigestive microbiome by antibiotic use, may influence future recommendations regarding therapy. Complementary and alternative medicine for OME and AOM have not been adequately studied and would require many enrolled subjects, standardized quality and dosing of the CAM therapy, and placebo or comparative head-to-head study design. Studies using current, most stringent criteria for diagnosis of AOM may find greater benefit for placement of tympanostomy tubes in recurrent AOM with or without MEE.

The FDA recently approved balloon dilation of Eustachian tubes for patients 22 years and older with chronic ETD (recurrent acute infections, chronic ME infection, or OME) based on obvious benefit over nasal steroid spray control in a randomized clinical trial of almost 300 patients.[55,56] The applicability of this novel technology to younger patients with chronic or complicated ETD, who have not responded to first-line surgical therapies, is yet to be determined, but preliminary studies in Europe regarding ballooning of ET in children seem to show promise.

SUMMARY

Nearly all preschool-age children are affected by AOM and/or OME. This article reviewed the pathophysiology of ETD and recent CPG available to guide the accurate diagnosis and evidence-based management of pediatric otitis media, with the goal of better aligning the practice patterns of clinicians who routinely care for pediatric patients.

REFERENCES

1. Shekelle P, Takata G, Chan LS, et al. Diagnosis, natural history and late effects of otitis media with effusion: evidence report/technology assessment no 55. Rockville (MD): Agency for Healthcare Research and Quality; 2003. AHRQ publication 03–E023.

2. Centers for Disease Control and Prevention. Table 2: top 5 diagnoses at visits to office-based physicians and hospital outpatient departments by patient age and sex: United States 2008. In: National ambulatory health care survey 2008. Atlanta (GA): Centers for Disease Control and Prevention; 2008.

3. Vernacchio L, Vezina RM, Mitchell AA. Management of acute otitis media by primary care physicians: trends since the release of the 2004 AAP/AAFP clinical practice guideline. Pediatrics 2007;120(2):281–7.
4. Forrest CB, Fiks AG, Bailey LC, et al. Improving adherence to otitis media guidelines with clinical decision support and physician feedback. Pediatrics 2013;131: e1071–81.
5. Lannon C, Peterson LE, Goudie A. Quality measures for the care of children with otitis media with effusion. Pediatrics 2011;127:e1409–97.
6. Rosenfeld RM, Culpepper L, Doyle KJ, et al. Clinical practice guideline: otitis media with effusion. Otolaryngol Head Neck Surg 2004;130(5):S95–118.
7. Mandel EM, Doyle WJ, Winter B, et al. The incidence, prevalence and burden of OM in unselected children aged 1-8 years followed by weekly otoscopy through the "common cold" season. Int J Pediatr Otorhinolaryngol 2008;72:491–9.
8. Tos M. Epidemiology and natural history of secretory otitis. Am J Otol 1984;5: 459–62.
9. Todberg T, Koch A, Andersson M, et al. Incidence of otitis media in a contemporary Danish National Birth Cohort. PLoS One 2014;9:e111732.
10. Walker RE, Bartley J, Flint D, et al. Determinants of chronic otitis media with effusion in preschool children: a case-control study. BMC Pediatr 2017;17(1):4.
11. Stool SE, Berg AO, Berman S, et al. Otitis media with effusion in young children: clinical practice guideline no. 12. Rockville (MD): Agency for Healthcare Research and Quality; 1994. AHCPR publication 94–0622.
12. Williamson I. Otitis media with effusion. Clin Evid 2002;7:469–76.
13. Casselbrant ML, Madel EM. Epidemiology. In: Rosenfeld RM, Bluestone CD, editors. Evidence-based otitis media. 2nd edition. Hamilton (Canada): BC Decker Inc; 2003. p. 147–62.
14. Martines F, Bentivenga D, Di Piazza F, et al. The point prevalence of otitis media with effusion among primary school children in Western Sicily. Eur Arch Otorhinolaryngol 2010;267:709–14.
15. Rosenfeld RM, Kay D. Natural history of untreated otitis media. Laryngoscope 2003;113:1645–57.
16. Brouwer CN, Maillé AR, Rovers MM, et al. Health-related quality of life in children with otitis media. Int J Pediatr Otorhinolaryngol 2005;69:1031–41.
17. Monasta L, Ronfani L, Marchetti F, et al. Burden of disease caused by otitis media: systematic review and global estimates. PLoS One 2012;7:336226.
18. Rovers MM. The burden of otitis media. Vaccine 2008;26(suppl 7):G2–4.
19. Qureishi A, Lee Y, Belfield K, et al. Update on otitis media: prevention and treatment. Infect Drug Resist 2014;7:15–24.
20. Timmerman AA, Anteunis LJC, Meesters CMG. Response-shift bias and parent-reported QOL in children with otitis media. Arch Otolaryngol Head Neck Surg 2003;129:987–91.
21. Zhou F, Shefer A, Kong Y, et al. Trends in acute otitis media-related health care utilization by privately insured young children in the United States, 1997-2004. Pediatrics 2008;121:253–60.
22. Maron T, Tan A, Wilkinson GS, et al. Trends in otitis media-related health care use in the United States, 2001-20011. JAMA Pediatr 2014;168:68–75.
23. Alsarraf R, Jung CJ, Perkins J, et al. Measuring the indirect and direct costs of acute otitis media. Arch Otolaryngol Head Neck Surg 1999;125:12–8.
24. Paradise JL, Bernard BS, Colborn DK. Pittsburgh-area Child Development/Otitis Media Study Group. Otitis media with effusion: highly prevalent and often the

forerunner of acute otitis media during the first year of life. Pediatr Res 1993;33: 121A.

25. Liberthal A, Carroll A, Chonmaitree T, et al. The diagnosis and management of acute otitis media. Pediatrics 2013;131(3):e964–99.

26. Rosenfeld RM, Shin J, Schwartz S, et al. Clinical practice guideline: otitis media with effusion (update). Otolaryngol Head Neck Surg 2016;154(IS):S1–41.

27. Boudewyns A, Declau F, Van den Ende J, et al. Otitis media with effusion: an underestimated cause of hearing loss in infants. Otol Neurotol 2011;32:799–804.

28. Rosenfeld RM, Schwartz SR, Pynnonen MA, et al. Clinical practice guideline: tympanostomy tubes in children. Otolaryngol Head Neck Surg 2013;149(1):S1–35.

29. Bhutta MF. Epidemiology and pathogenesis of otitis media: construction of phenotype landscape. Audiol Neurootol 2014;19:210–23.

30. van Balen F, de Melker RA. Persistent otitis media with effusion: can it be predicted? A family practice follow-up study in children aged 6 months to 6 years. J Fam Pract 2000;49:605–11.

31. Cullen KA, Hall MJ, Golosinskiy A. Ambulatory surgery in the United States, 2006. Natl Health Stat Rep 2009;(11):1–25.

32. Mui S, Rasgon BM, Hilsinger RL Jr, et al. Tympanostomy tubes for otitis media: quality-of-life improvement for children and parents. Ear Nose Throat J 2005; 84(7):418, 420–412, 424.

33. Kay DJ, Nelson M, Rosenfeld RM. Meta-analysis of tympanostomy tube sequelae. Otolaryngol Head Neck Surg 2001;124(4):374–80.

34. Granath A, Rynnel-Dagoo B, Backheden M, et al. Tube-associated otorrhea in children with recurrent acute otitis media; results of a prospective, randomized study on bacteriology and topical treatment with or without systemic antibiotics. Int J Pediatr Otorhinolaryngol 2008;72(8):1225–33.

35. Rothman R, Owens T, Simel DL. Does this child have acute otitis media? JAMA 2003;290(12):1633–40.

36. Laine MK, Tähtinen PA, Ruuskanen O, et al. Symptoms or symptom-based scores cannot predict acute otitis media at otitis-prone age. Pediatrics 2010;125(5): e1154–61.

37. Shaikh N, Hoberman A, Paradise JL, et al. Responsiveness and construct validity of a symptom scale for acute otitis media. Pediatr Infect Dis J 2009;28(1):9–12.

38. Rovers MM, Glasziou P, Appelman CL, et al. Predictors of pain and/or fever at 3 to 7 days for children with acute otitis media not treated initially with antibiotics: a metanalysis of individual patient data. Pediatrics 2007;119(3):579–85.

39. Sanders S, Glasziou PP, Del Mar C. Antibiotics for acute otitis media in children (review). Cochrane Database Syst Rev 2009;(2):1–43.

40. American Academy of Pediatrics. Committee on Psychosocial Aspects of Child and Family Health, Task Force on Pain in Infants, Children, and Adolescents. The assessment and management of acute pain in infants, children and adolescents. Pediatrics 2001;108(3):793–7.

41. Bolt P, Barnett P, Babl FE, et al. Topical lidocane for pain relief in acute otitis media: results of a double-blind placebo-controlled randomized trial. Arch Dis Child 2008;93(1):40–4.

42. Mujica-Mota MA, Bezdjian A, Salehi P, et al. Assessment of ototoxicity of intratympanic administration of Auralgan in a chinchilla animal model. Laryngoscope 2015;125(6):1444–8.

43. Available at: https://www.fda.gov/Safety/MedWatch/SafetyInformation/Safety AlertsforHumanMedicalProducts/ucm453430.htm. Accessed June 23, 2017.

44. Heikkinen T, Chonmaitree T. Importance of respiratory viruses in acute otitis media. Clin Microbiol Rev 2003;16(2):230–41.
45. Rosenfeld RM, Vertrees J, Carr J, et al. Clinical efficacy of antimicrobials for acute otitis media: meta-analysis of 5,400 children from 33 randomized trials. J Pediatr 1994;124(3):355–67.
46. Piglansky L, Leibovitz E, Raiz S, et al. Bacteriologic and clinical efficacy of high dose amoxicillin for therapy of acute otitis media in children. Pediatr Infect Dis J 2003;22(5):405–13.
47. Pichichero ME. Use of selected cephalosporins in penicillin-allergic patients: a paradigm shift. Diagn Microbiol Infect Dis 2007;57(suppl 3):13S–8S.
48. Leibovitz E, Piglansky L, Raiz S, et al. Bateriologic and clinical efficacy of one day vs. three day intramuscular ceftriaxone for treatment of nonresponsive acute otitis media in children. Pediatr Infect Dis J 2000;19(11):1040–5.
49. Kozyrskj AL, Klassen TP, Moffatt M, et al. Short-course antibiotics for acute otitis media. Cochrane Database Syst Rev 2010;(9):CD001095.
50. McCormick DP, Chonmaitree T, Pittman C, et al. Nonsevere acute otitis media: a clinical trial comparing outcomes of watchful waiting versus immediate antibiotic treatment. Pediatrics 2005;115(6):1455–65.
51. Little P, Gould C, Williamson I, et al. Pragmatic randomized controlled trial of two prescribing strategies for childhood acute otitis media. BMJ 2001;322(7282):336–42.
52. Leach AJ, Morris PS. Antibiotics for the prevention of acute and chronic suppurative otitis media in children. Cochrane Database Syst Rev 2006;(4):CD004401.
53. Hellstrom S, Groth A, Jorgensent F, et al. Ventilation tube treatment: a systematic review of the literature. Otolaryngol Head Neck Surg 2011;145(3):383–95.
54. McDonald S, Langton Hewer CD, Nunez DA. Grommets (ventilation tubes) for recurrent acute otitis media in children. Cochrane Database Syst Rev 2008;(4):CD004741.
55. Food and Drug Administration, HHS. Medical devices; ear, nose, and throat devices; classification of the eustachian tube balloon dilation system. Final order. Fed Regist 2016;81(205):73028–30.
56. Poe D. In reference to balloon dilatation eustachian tuboplasty: a clinical study. Laryngoscope 2011;121(5):908.

Cochlear Implants in the Elderly
Recognizing a Frequently Missed Demographic of Surgical Candidates for Hearing Restoration

Holly J. Baker, MHS, PA-C[a,b,]*, Robert T. Sataloff, MD, DMA[c]

KEYWORDS

- Cochlear implants • Presbycusis • Conventional hearing aids
- Age-related hearing loss • Hearing amplification • Speech discrimination

KEY POINTS

- Cochlear implants may be an attractive option for elderly patients diagnosed with hearing impairments who no longer benefit from conventional hearing aids.
- Cochlear implants differ from conventional hearing aids in that they not only improve communication, but deliver adequate amplification to improve word understanding and speech discrimination.
- Elderly patients should be educated about evolving candidacy criteria, benefits on speech and overall quality of life, and the minimal risk associated with the procedure.
- Providers have a responsibility to inform patients of all treatment options, including cochlear implants.

HEARING LOSS: AN OVERVIEW

Hearing loss remains a major public health issue in the United States and is ranked third after arthritis and heart disease.[1] Hearing loss can affect people of all ages, varies in progression from mild to profound loss, and is caused by several different etiologies. The hearing pathway is a complex pathway that changes sound waves into electrical signals sent to the auditory nerve that carries these signals to the brain. Sound waves enter the outer ear and travel through the ear canal to the eardrum. The sound waves cause vibration of the eardrum, which sends the

No Disclosures.
[a] Otolaryngology–Head and Neck Surgery, ENT and Allergy Specialists, 825 Old Lancaster Road, Suite 300, Bryn Mawr, PA 19010, USA; [b] Department of Otolaryngology–Head and Neck Surgery, Drexel University College of Medicine, 2900 West Queen Lane, Philadelphia, PA 19129, USA; [c] Department of Otolaryngology–Head and Neck Surgery, Drexel University College of Medicine, 219 North Broad Street, 10th Floor, Philadelphia, PA 19107, USA
* Corresponding author. 219 N. Broad Street The Arnold T. Berman, MD Building, 10th Floor Philadelphia, PA 19107.
E-mail address: HJP1487@gmail.com

Physician Assist Clin 3 (2018) 223–234
https://doi.org/10.1016/j.cpha.2017.12.004
2405-7991/18/© 2017 Elsevier Inc. All rights reserved.

vibrations to the bony ossicles within the middle ear (malleus, incus, and stapes). Vibrations from the ossicles are transmitted into the fluid-filled cochlea known as the inner ear, stimulating the cochlear hair cells, which generate electrical signals for the auditory nerve.

The 3 types of hearing loss are sensorineural, conductive, and mixed hearing loss. Sensorineural hearing loss is described as a "nerve loss" and can result from damage to parts of the inner ear, the auditory nerve, or cerebral hearing processing. Sensorineural hearing loss can also be caused by prolonged exposure to loud noise, head injury, infection, prescription drugs, and many other etiologies.[2,3] Rates of progression vary, and this type of hearing loss generally cannot be medically or surgically restored at this time. Conductive hearing loss is described as a "bone conduction" loss and occurs when sound is not conducted efficiently through the outer or middle ear structures. Conductive hearing loss can be caused by fluid in the middle ear, otitis media, allergies, Eustachian tube dysfunction, perforated eardrum, benign tumors of the middle ear, cerumen impaction, foreign body obstructing the ear canal, or malformation of the outer ear, ear canal, or middle ear. Conductive causes of hearing loss can often be corrected medically or surgically. Last, mixed hearing loss is a combination of sensorineural hearing loss and conductive hearing loss[2] (**Fig. 1**).

SENSORINEURAL HEARING LOSS AND THE ELDERLY POPULATION

According to the National Institutes of Health, approximately 15% of American adults (37.5 million) aged 18 years and over report some degree of hearing loss. With age being the strongest predictor of hearing loss among adults aged 20 to 69 years, those with the greatest amount of hearing loss fall in the range of 60 to 69 years of age.[4] Given the aging population of Baby Boomers in the United States and

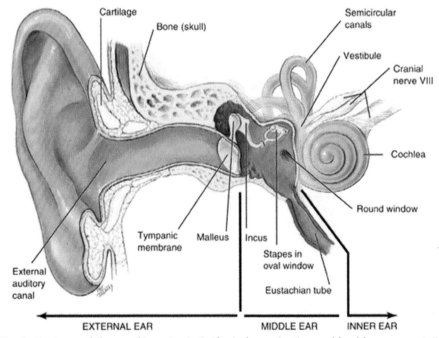

Fig. 1. Anatomy of the ear. (*From* Jarvis C. Physical examination and health assessment. 5 edition. Philadelphia: Saunders-Elsevier; 2008; with permission.)

increasing of life expectancy, the absolute number of persons impacted by hearing loss is expected to increase in the coming years. Within the hearing impaired population, there is an overwhelming gap in the number of individuals using hearing devices and those who are not. In fact, among adults aged 70 years and older with hearing loss who could benefit from hearing aids, fewer than 30% have ever used them.[4] Over the past decade, many have questioned contributors to this significant disparity between device users and nonusers, because there have been substantial advancements in the rehabilitation of hearing loss.

At the present time, 50% to 60% of today's elderly population over 70 years of age experiences some form of hearing loss.[5] Presbycusis remains the most common cause of hearing loss in the elderly. Presbycusis, also known as age-related hearing loss, is sensorineural in nature and typically presents with a slow decline in hearing. Hearing impairments affect both speech perception and speech production. This, in turn, has a negative impact on social interactions, often leading to social isolation and decreased employment opportunities, which may lead to lost income and a decrease in quality of life.[6] Additionally, patient safety relating to automobile, occupational, environmental, and other hazards is a concern for the hearing impaired, because these individuals cannot appropriately receive the auditory stimuli as alerts to presence of danger. The work of Benatti and colleagues[5] has also concluded that hearing loss is associated with a 2- to 5-fold increased risk for developing dementia, as well as a 1.4 times greater odds of having a fall.

TRADITIONAL AMPLIFICATION WITH HEARING AIDS

Among the hearing impaired, the elderly present with a combination of age-related central and peripheral degenerative changes in all sensorineural processes, including the auditory system. Traditional hearing aids do not provide adequate amplification to those with advanced hearing loss. Hearing aids can improve communication in most individuals, but in the case of severe to profound loss, they are unable to produce adequate amplification and fail to improve the individual's word discrimination and speech understanding[6] (**Fig. 2**).

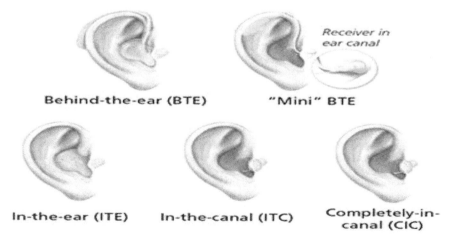

Behind-the-ear (BTE)

Receiver in ear canal

"Mini" BTE

In-the-ear (ITE)

In-the-canal (ITC)

Completely-in-canal (CIC)

Fig. 2. Examples of traditional hearing aids. (*Courtesy of* The National Institutes of Health, Department of Health and Human Services, Bethesda, MD; and *Data from* Hearing aids. National Institute on Deafness and Other Communication Disorders (NIDCD). 2013. Available at: https://www.nidcd.nih.gov/health/hearing-aids. Accessed August 14, 2017.)

Speech discrimination entails the patient's ability to accurately discern different spoken words; as the percentage of correct responses during auditory testing decreases, so does the benefit of conventional hearing aids. When speech discrimination score is 100%, an individual will understand everything heard; if the speech recognition score is 0%, one does not understand any words spoken, no matter how loud the speech is presented. Those with a good speech recognition score (≥80%) would find traditional hearing aids useful. However, those with a very poor speech recognition score (<40%) would receive no benefit from traditional hearing aids and often find the sound coming in muffled and undiscernible.[7] Those with a speech recognition score in the 60% to 70% range may or may not find hearing aids useful, and many audiologists may provide a trial of amplification to this subset of patients. When a patient experiences little benefit from conventional hearing aids, other hearing rehabilitation options should be offered, including surgically implanted auditory devices such as cochlear implants (**Box 1**).

Box 1
Word recognition score by percent

Speech discrimination score

90% to 100% = excellent

78% to 88% = good or slight difficulty

66% to 76% = fair or moderate difficulty

54% to 64% = poor or great difficulty

Less than 52% = very poor

Data from Schoepflin J. Back to basics: speech audiometry. Audiology online. 2012. Available at: http://www.audiologyonline.com/articles/back-to-basics-speech-audiometry-6828. Accessed August 13, 2017.

AURAL REHABILITATION THROUGH COCHLEAR IMPLANTATION

In the past decade, the use of hearing devices such as cochlear implants has increased in popularity in patients who no longer receive sufficient benefit from conventional hearing aid(s). Cochlear implants are now available to patients with varying degrees of hearing loss and restore hearing through internal and external components that work together to allow the user to perceive sound. The external portion, consisting of a microphone, speech processer, and transmitter, sends a coded signal to the implanted receiver underneath the skin. The receiver delivers the signal to electrodes that have been embedded into the cochlea, which stimulate the fibers of the auditory nerve, thereby activating auditory pathways in the brain[8] (**Fig. 3**).

COCHLEAR IMPLANTATION: SURGERY AND REHABILITATION

Cochlear implant surgery is performed under general anesthesia and patients with significant medical comorbidity should have a prior anesthetic risk assessment. The surgery typically takes between 1 and 2 hours to complete, and patients are likely discharged the same day or on postoperative day 1. Before surgery, it is important to confirm a clear middle ear space through otoscopy, tympanometry, and/or temporal bone imaging. This step ensures that there is no active infection, to avoid the implant serving as a conduit to deep, even intracranial, infection. A postauricular incision is used and the surgical approach involves a standard

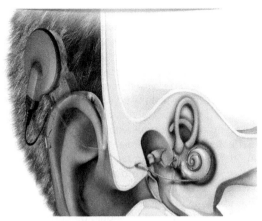

Fig. 3. Cochlear implant. (*Courtesy of* Med El, Durham, NC; and *Data from* Med El. Available at: http://www.medel.com/us/. Accessed August 16, 2017.)

mastoidectomy and cochleostomy where electrode arrays are inserted near or communicating with the round window into the cochlea. Once the device is implanted and the wound closed, telemetry programs are activated, which measure electrode impedances and action potentials important for identifying open circuits.[9]

Perioperative and postoperative complications are fortunately uncommon with cochlear implantation. With advancements in surgical implants and techniques, both medical and surgical complications have become rare. Medical and surgical complications were historically far more common compared with device-related issues, primarily due to the fact that postauricular incisions were larger, devices were more rigid, and device placement was closer to the mastoid cavity.[9] Common perioperative complications include taste disturbance owing to damage to the chorda tympani nerve (which travels through the middle ear space), transient dizziness, hemotympanum, and subcutaneous seroma. Other complications involving the device itself include internal device failure (ie, dead device), internal suspected malfunction, speech processor failure, accessory malfunction, and open electrode circuits. Although complications relating to the device may occur, cochlear implant revision surgery results in a functioning device in most instances (**Box 2**).[9]

Additional research supports the position that neither age nor the risk of surgical complications should not automatically disqualify elderly patients from receiving cochlear implants. Postoperative complications were examined in a number of studies focused on older adults, namely, those over 60 years of age, with a mean age of

Box 2	
Complications of cochlear implantation	
Medical or Surgical	**Device Related**
Taste disturbance	Internal failure (dead device)
Dizziness	Internal suspected malfunction
Subcutaneous seroma	Speech processor failure
Dural or vascular injury	Accessory malfunction
Flap or wound infection	Open electrode circuits

Data from Johnson JT, Rosen CA. Bailey's head and neck surgery: otolaryngology. vol. 2. 5th edition. Baltimore (MD): Lippincott Williams & Wilkin; 2014; with permission.

72 years. These studies demonstrated that vestibular symptoms such as dizziness and vertigo after implantation were nonexistent.[10,11] Furthermore, postoperative infection, facial weakness, flap dehiscence, and balance issues were noted in less than 5% of those patients at 5 and 10 years after implantation.[10,11] These results support the notion that concerns for increased postoperative complications in the older patient population need not be a primary deterrent when determining candidacy.

Receiving a cochlear implant is a lifetime commitment and outcomes depend heavily on appropriate expectations among patients and their families. After surgery, follow-up visits entail fitting of the external components, activating and programming the implant and its accessories, any necessary adjustments and reprogramming, and annual checkups. In addition to follow-up care, recipients may require aural rehabilitation. Aural rehabilitation programs have been shown to significantly improve outcomes and provide faster progress in learning to accurately identify sounds and ability to comprehend speech.[12] If implanted patients have difficulty with any of the following, some form of aural rehabilitation should be considered:

- Understanding most speakers easily and completely;
- Understanding a speaker without seeing his or her face or at a distance;
- Speech comprehension in both loud and quiet environments;
- Participating in group discussions;
- Using the telephone; and
- Anxiety in new environments owing to fear of communicating.

Rehabilitation entails several different therapeutic approaches, including auditory therapy, speech therapy, repair strategy training, environmental manipulation, telephone training, and music appreciation training. There is variability as to the frequency and type of rehabilitation adults may benefit from with a cochlear implant.[12]

INDICATIONS AND CRITERIA FOR COCHLEAR IMPLANTATION

The precise number of individuals who might benefit from a cochlear implant has been estimated by a number of sources. Of the 50% to 60% of the US population over 70 years of age, a substantial number of those with hearing loss can no longer benefit from a conventional hearing aid.[5,13] It has been estimated that 0.6% to 1.1% of hearing impaired patients have a severe to profound hearing loss and receive little to no benefit from using traditional hearing aids.[5] Although studies indicate a wide range of possibility for how many elderly individuals in the United States are potential candidates, the American Speech-Language Hearing Association reports that anywhere from 250,000 to 1 million persons may benefit from cochlear implantation, and that number is expected to increase over the coming years with the aging of the US population.[14]

With the number of candidates for cochlear implants increasing, it is important to discuss who qualifies for candidacy. However, there is no straightforward answer to who meets the criteria for a cochlear implantation. Since cochlear implant was approved by the US Food and Drug Administration in 1985 and 1990, for adult and pediatric use, respectively, the criteria for implantation have evolved dramatically. In 1985, only adults diagnosed with postlinguistic, profound hearing loss with 0% aided speech discrimination scores were approved for cochlear implantation.[15] Today, implantation criteria span the age range from infant to geriatric, and include those with a lesser degree of hearing loss and higher speech discrimination scores. Therefore, patients who suffer from only moderate sloping toward profound loss may still be excellent candidates for a cochlear implantation (See Table 1 – Criteria for implant by

Cochlear Americas: 1985 versus present at: https://www.audiologyonline.com/articles/unidentified-and-underserved-cochlear-implant-876).

Cochlear implant candidacy also varies among implant manufacturers and insurance carriers. For example, with respect to the degree of hearing loss and audiometric thresholds, two implant manufacturers, Advanced Bionics (Stäfa, Switzerland) and Med El (Durham, NC), specify bilateral "severe" (61–80 dB) to "profound" (81 dB or greater) sensorineural hearing loss for adult implant candidacy, whereas another manufacturer, Cochlear Americas (Centennial, CO), specifies bilateral "moderate" (41–60 dB) to "profound" (≥81 dB) loss.[16]

All potential candidates require comprehensive neurotologic evaluation to detect or rule out serious and treatable etiologies for hearing loss.[2] As part of the implant process, a preimplant evaluation answers common questions including surgical and postoperative process, follow-up and intervention schedules, cost, realistic expectations, warranties, and insurance coverage. An audiological evaluation is performed to confirm whether or not amplification with high-powered hearing aids can or cannot provide enough auditory information. A medical evaluation by the surgeon will determine general anesthesia risks and medical comorbidities. The surgical consultation also includes an in-depth discussion with the patient and family to develop an understanding of the benefits and limitations of a cochlear implant, as well as reasonable expectations after implantation. In certain circumstances, an assessment of psychological factors can be useful before implantation. Temporal bone imaging is critical in all recipients to identify the etiology of hearing loss, and to define surgical anatomy and any potential complications or sequelae including developmental labyrinthine conditions, cochlear nerve deficiency, otosclerosis, inflammation, fibrosis, or ossification of the inner ear (**Box 3**).[9]

There are few absolute contraindications for cochlear implantation. Patients with an absent cochlea (Michel aplasia) or cochlear nerve are not candidates for surgery. Relative contraindications include active middle ear disease and severe anesthetic risk. Patients with an expected lower level of performance owing to cochlear disorders and/or auditory nerve disorders (including obstruction from previous meningitis, otosclerosis, severe inner ear malformation with cochlear nerve deficiency, and vestibular schwannoma) may require more detailed preoperative counseling. Additionally, any damage to the central nervous system owing to prior stroke or degenerative diseases (ie, multiple sclerosis, dementia) should be uncovered preoperatively, because these conditions may limit benefit from implantation. Although cochlear disorders, auditory nerve disorders, and damage to the central nervous system should lower expectations and may reduce the benefits of implantation, it is important to note that these are not contraindications to the cochlear implant surgery itself.[9]

Box 3 Grades of hearing loss		
Grade	**dB**	**Description**
Mild	26–40	Difficulty with soft speech, speech at a distance, and with background noise
Moderate	41–60	Difficulty with regular speech at normal distance
Severe	61–80	Difficulty with most conversational speech and may only hear very loud speech and sounds
Profound	>81	May only perceive loud sounds as vibrations

Adapted from Grades of hearing impairment. World Health Organization. Available at: http://www.who.int/pbd/deafness/hearing_impairment_grades/en/. Accessed May 31, 2017; with permission.

THE BENEFITS OF COCHLEAR IMPLANTATION IN THE ELDERLY POPULATION

Given the substantial number of individuals who meet cochlear implant candidacy criteria, and the incidence of hearing impairment with age, the benefits of implants in the elderly population have been researched in several studies. Numerous studies discuss how patients with implants have the opportunity for significant improvements in speech recognition and speech production, and indicate that elders can gain outstanding results after cochlear implant, even though they may require more counseling and attention.[5,17] For example, individuals with significant hearing loss often rely on visual cues such as lip reading for communication. This dependence can be completely or nearly eliminated with the use of an implant.[5]

Cochlear implants also improve speech reading by providing auditory information on prosody. Several studies' results indicated that there was significant improvement after cochlear implant in pure tone hearing thresholds as well as speech discrimination, comparable with that of young adult implanted users.[10,18,19] One study concluded that there was nearly 50% improvement in audiological and speech understanding performances from preoperative to postoperative in elderly implanted patients.[19] Further research has implicated hearing loss in the development of social isolation.[20] Auditory rehabilitation such as cochlear implant promotes social engagement in older persons through improved communication abilities, leading to an overall improvement in quality of life.[20]

PATIENT EDUCATION: HEARING LOSS AND TREATMENT OPTIONS

Given the substantial benefits and minimal risk associated with the procedure itself, cochlear implants should undeniably be recommended to elderly patients who meet the current criteria. Patients frequently turn to their primary care providers as their principal point of contact for medical concerns, including hearing loss. Medical professionals should have an understanding of cochlear implants and be well-equipped to recognize, educate, and refer suitable patients appropriately. It is a shared responsibility among providers to advise patients of all treatment options that might be in their best interest, and those who lack an understanding of cochlear implants risk undertreating or missing eligible patients.

Several studies done in the past decade have shown that there is, in fact, an absence of awareness by medical professionals of the current cochlear implant candidacy criteria.[21–23] Not only is there a lack of knowledge regarding cochlear implant, study results also have shown a steady decrease in the number of routine annual hearing screens. One study in 2005 surveyed 80,000 members of the National Family Opinion panel, which consists of households that are balanced to the latest US census information with respect to market size, age of household, and income.[21] Investigators specifically asked individuals who had received their general medical examination within the last 6 months to indicate if their provider had performed a hearing screening. Results showed that hearing evaluation rate had decreased to 12.9% from 18.0% for the total population and decreases in screening were seen in every age group except young adults.[21] Cohen and colleagues[22] and Danhauer and associates[23] reported similar data, concluding that 60% of physicians surveyed reported that they did not routinely screen for hearing loss owing to a "lack of time" and "more pressing issues." Huart[15] also found similar results in a survey taken at the AudiologyNOW! Conference in Charlotte, North Carolina, where attendees including practitioners and audiologists responded to a questionnaire regarding the identification and referral of patients for cochlear implant evaluation. Before the conference and learning candidacy criteria, 20% of audiologists surveyed believed they had not seen any potential candidate in their office in the last 6 months, and 55% responded that they had seen fewer than 5 patients, resulting in a combined 75% of those who took the survey believing that they had examined fewer than 5 patients in their practice who might be a prospective recipient for an implant in the prior 6 months. When asked about referral, more than 90% had referred fewer than 5 patients for a cochlear implant evaluation.[15]

When comparing these survey results with the statistical on the large number of potential cochlear implant candidates in the United States, the number of identified potential cochlear implant candidates seems surprisingly low.[15] Given these statistics, it seems only rational that, if medical professionals are not cognizant of the criteria, benefits, and other basic information supporting cochlear implantation, they cannot successfully identify potential candidates. Cochlear Americas conducted a similar survey in which implant recipients were asked who referred them for their initial implant evaluation. Not surprisingly, fewer than one-half were referred by audiologists and nearly 20% reported they were not referred by any type of health care professional; instead, they had learned about the possibility of cochlear implant through friends, family, or the Internet.

In a large, multicenter, clinical study, it was discovered that the average time from progression to severe hearing loss to receiving an implant was 12 years.[24] This study supports the fact that there is indeed a "disconnect" between medical professionals and cochlear implant candidates, and confirms that medical professionals could be doing a better job of identifying potential implant candidates. The study also illustrates that, once hearing impaired individuals became aware of their candidacy, there was often very little hesitation to proceed. In fact, 1500 recipients were surveyed, and results found that most had received their implant less than 1 year after determination that they met candidacy criteria.[15] If medical professionals recommended a routine hearing screening in elderly patients, gained a better understanding regarding cochlear implant candidacy criteria, and were familiarized with the benefits of cochlear implantation, then these providers could properly identify, educate, and refer prospective patients sooner.

Cochlear implants have been increasing in popularity and have become a valuable option for the hearing impaired population. According to the National Institute on Deafness and Other Communication Disorders, as of December 2012, approximately 324,200 people worldwide have received cochlear implants.[25] In the United States, it is estimated that 58,000 adults (60% of recipients) and 38,000 children (40%) have received an implant.[25] However, Huart[15] explains that, "even though the absolute percentage is higher in adults, the ratio of recipients to candidates is lower for adults than for children because hearing loss is more common in adults."

Even though hearing loss is considered one of the most common sensory impairments, this deficit has been largely neglected in the field of public health. With a shared responsibility among providers to recognize difficulties in hearing, future research should be focused on educating both patients and providers regarding hearing loss and treatment options. The World Health Organization (WHO) assists in developing programs for ear and hearing care that are integrated into the primary health care system. In addition, the WHO provides technical resources and guidance for training health care professionals on hearing loss and advocates for awareness about the prevalence, causes, and impact of hearing loss as well as prevention, identification, and management.[26] However, small journals aimed at primary care providers and/or hearing specialists may help providers to recognize and diagnose hearing loss earlier, as well as identify which hearing impaired patients may be cochlear implant candidates. Also, as with any health-related concern, prevention is important. Educating the general public on the preventable risk factors for hearing loss (including ototoxic medications; infections such as measles, meningitis and mumps; and noise exposure) may decrease the overall incidence of hearing loss. Last, educational efforts should continue to highlight the association between the benefits of cochlear implants in the elderly population and overall improvements in hearing and speech, as well as quality of life.

AREAS FOR FUTURE RESEARCH

Although traditional hearing aids and cochlear implants remain the mainstay of treatment for sensorineural hearing loss, there have been continued efforts in medical technology advancements and new medical discoveries. The candidacy criteria for cochlear implants will continue to evolve over time and other approaches for hearing restoration are actively being explored. Areas for future research involving the pursuit of regenerative treatments for sensorineural hearing loss include gene transfer, pharmacotherapies, exogenous delivery of stem cells, and the promotion of endogenous stem cells.[27] Each potential therapy entails unique challenges, including safe and efficient methods to access the cochlea, repopulating the cochlea with a sufficient number of cells, avoidance of generating hair cells outside the organ of corti, maintenance of newly generated cells, and the reestablishment of neuronal circuitry.[27] Although to date these approaches remain in the experimental stages with no clinical trials in adults, numerous laboratories worldwide continue to remain actively involved in this promising area of research.

SUMMARY

The number of elderly patients who would benefit from a cochlear implant is already astoundingly high, and research estimates this number will continue to increase in the coming years. By recognizing potential candidates for implantation early and proceeding with careful evaluation, referral for timely cochlear implantation shows great promise in lessening the negative impact of hearing loss on patients' quality of life. Furthermore, the benefits of cochlear implant undoubtedly outweigh the risks for most patients. The substantial gap between users and nonusers of hearing devices, including cochlear implants, presents a challenge to the medical profession. Those who no longer benefit from a conventional hearing aid often give up on this modality, and it is up to medical professionals to educate these patients on further treatment options available. If medical professionals recommended routine hearing screenings, were better educated about hearing loss, and were equipped to discuss all auditory rehabilitation options, including cochlear implants, the gap between users and nonusers of hearing devices should decrease. Last, and most important, patients who are equipped with enhanced knowledge and diagnostics regarding their hearing loss would have the opportunity to avail themselves of the benefits of improved communication and a better quality of life, which can be provided by cochlear implants and other auditory rehabilitation devices.

REFERENCES

1. Basic facts about hearing loss. Hearing loss association of America. Available at: http://www.hearingloss.org/content/basic-facts-about-hearing-loss. Accessed August 14, 2017.
2. Sataloff RT, Sataloff J. Hearing loss. 4th edition. New York: Taylor and Francis; 2005.
3. Netter FH. Atlas of human anatomy. 4th edition. Philadelphia: Saunders Elsevier; 2006.

4. Quick statistics about hearing. National Institute on Deafness and Other Communication Disorders (NIDCD). 2016. Available at: https://www.nidcd.nih.gov/health/statistics/quick-statistics-hearing#3. Accessed May 31, 2017.

5. Benatti A, Montino S, Girasoli L, et al. Cochlear implantation in the elderly: surgical and hearing outcomes. BMC Surg 2013;13(Suppl 2):S1.

6. Migirov L, Taitelbaum-Swead R, Drendel M, et al. Cochlear implantation in elderly patients: surgical and audiological outcome. Gerontology 2010;56(2):123–8.

7. Bauman N. What is speech discrimination? Center for hearing loss help. 2017. http://hearinglosshelp.com/blog/what-is-speech-discrimination/. Accessed August 14, 2017.

8. Cochlear implants. American Speech-Language Hearing Association (ASHA). 2014. Available at: http://www.asha.org/public/hearing/Cochlear-Implant/. Accessed May 22, 2017.

9. Johnson JT, Rosen CA. 5th edition. Bailey's head and neck surgery: otolaryngology, vol. 2. Baltimore (MD): Lippincott Williams & Wilkin; 2014.

10. Roberts DS, Lin HW, Hermann BS, et al. Differential cochlear implant outcomes in older adults. Laryngoscope 2013;123(8):1952–6.

11. Chen DS, Clarrett DM, Li L, et al. Cochlear implantation in older adults: long-term analysis of complications and device survival in a consecutive series. Otol Neurotol 2013;34(7):1272–7.

12. Sorkin DL, Calaffe-Schenck M. Cochlear implant rehabilitation. It's not just for kids! Cochlear.com. 2008. Available at: http://www.cochlear.com/wps/wcm/connect/au/home/support/rehabilitation-resources/teens-and-adults. Accessed August 15, 2017.

13. Lin FR, Chien WW, Li L, et al. Cochlear implantation in older adults. Medicine (Baltimore) 2012;91(5):229–41.

14. Incidence and prevalence of hearing loss and hearing aid use in the United States. American Speech-Language Hearing Association (ASHA). Available at: www.asha.org/members/research/reports/hearing.htm. Accessed May 22, 2017.

15. Huart S. Unidentified and underserved: cochlear implant candidates in the hearing aid dispensing practice. Audiology online. 2009. Available at: http://www.audiologyonline.com/articles/unidentified-and-underserved-cochlear-implant-876. Accessed May 22, 2017.

16. Gifford RH. Who is a cochlear implant candidate? Hear J 2011;66(6):16, 18–22.

17. Filipo R, Ballantyne D, D'Elia C, et al. Cochlear implantation in elderly: indications and results. BMC Geriatr 2010;10(suppl 1):A107.

18. Sanchez-Cuadrado I, Lassaletta L, Perez-Mora RM, et al. Is there an age limit for cochlear implantation? Ann Otol Rhinol Laryngol 2013;122(4):222–8.

19. Lachowska M, Pastuszka A, Glinka P, et al. Is cochlear implantation a good treatment method for profoundly deafened elderly? Clin Interv Aging 2013;8:1339–46.

20. Mick P, Kawachi I, Lin F. The association between hearing loss and social isolation in older adults. Otolaryngol Head Neck Surg 2014;150(3):378–84.

21. Kochkin S. MarkeTrak VII: hearing loss population tops 31 million people. The Hearing Review 2005;12(7):16–29.

22. Cohen SM, Labadie RF, Haynes DS. Primary care approach to hearing loss: the hidden disability. Ear Nose Throat J 2005;84(1):26, 29–31, 44.

23. Danhauer JL, Celani KE, Johnson CE. Use of a hearing and balance screening survey with local primary care physicians. Am J Audiol 2008;17(1):3–13.

24. Balkany T, Hodges A, Menapace C, et al. Nucleus Freedom North American clinical trial. Otolaryngol Head Neck Surg 2007;136(5):757–62.

25. Cochlear implants. National Institute on Deafness and Other Communication Disorders (NIDCD). Available at: www.nidcd.nih.gov/health/hearing/coch.asp. Accessed May 22, 2017.

26. Media Centre. Deafness and hearing loss. Geneva, Switzerland: World Health Organization; 2017. Available at: http://www.who.int/mediacentre/factsheets/fs300/en/. Accessed August 15, 2017.

27. Sataloff RT, Johns MM, Kost KM. Geriatric otolaryngology. New York: Thieme; 2015.

Sudden Sensorineural Loss in Primary Care
An Often-Missed Diagnosis

Alan K. Mirly, MBA, PA-C[a],*, Jeff E. Brockett, EdD, CCC-A[b]

KEYWORDS

- Sudden sensorineural hearing loss • Intratympanic steroid • Primary care
- Sudden hearing loss

KEY POINTS

- Sudden sensorineural hearing loss (SSNHL) is commonly overlooked in primary care and may lead to permanent hearing loss.
- SSNHL should be differentiated from other types of hearing loss.
- Proper history and physical examination can help to identify SSNHL and may improve diagnosis of conductive losses.
- Most patients will initially present to primary care with sudden hearing loss. Identification of SSNHL and consideration for treatment should be made at the first visit.
- Treatment of SSNHL is a controversial topic without strong evidence that treatment offers significant improvement.

INTRODUCTION: A CASE OF SUDDEN HEARING LOSS

A healthy 56-year-old gentleman arrives in the provider's office on a Friday afternoon at 4:30 PM with report of sudden hearing loss.[1–3] He believes this started last night while he was helping his grandson with his homework. He states that he was having difficulty hearing his grandson with his right ear and heard a buzzing noise in the same ear. He assumed his grandson was not speaking clearly and he went to bed. This morning he answered the phone using his right ear as he typically does but could not make out anything. He has had some continued buzzing in the right ear with no improvement throughout the day. He also has a feeling of fullness in the right ear but denies vertigo. He denies any previous hearing loss and has had no recent or known prior noise trauma.

Disclosures: The authors have nothing to disclose.
[a] Pocatello Ear, Nose & Throat, Department of Physician Assistant Studies, Idaho State University, Pocatello, ID, USA; [b] Department of Communication Sciences and Disorders, Idaho State University, Pocatello, ID, USA
* Corresponding author.
E-mail address: mirlalan@isu.edu

This case represents a frequent dilemma faced by primary care providers and demonstrates a prototypical patient with an idiopathic sudden sensorineural hearing loss (ISSNHL). An ISSNHL can occur at any age; however peak incidence is the fifth and sixth decade, affecting men and women equally.[4] Fullness in the ear is almost always a presenting symptom and is commonly accompanied by tinnitus in 79%; vertigo in 31%[5]; and bilateral presentation, which is far less common, in 4.9% of cases.[6] The presenting concerns are the type of hearing loss, the best treatment options currently available, and what the patient should expect following this initial visit. The problem is that only 60% of primary care providers routinely assess for hearing loss,[7] indicating a potential clinical skills deficit and the impeding diagnosis of a potentially permanent sensory loss.

SUDDEN HEARING LOSS DEFINED

Sudden hearing loss is a generic term for hearing loss that occurs over a short time, typically less than 72 hours. A sudden sensorineural hearing loss (SSNHL) is most commonly defined as a hearing loss of 30 dB or greater at 3 consecutive frequencies,[8] occurring in less than 72 hours. Providers must first look for any underlying conditions that may account for the hearing loss. Retrocochlear processes, such as vestibular schwannomas or a stroke, account for less than 1% of cases, whereas other identifiable causes (eg, an inner ear disorder, trauma, infection, autoimmune disease, or ototoxic medication) account for 10% to 15%.[9] If no underlying conditions can be identified that account for the SSNHL, then providers can make the diagnosis of an ISSNHL.

ISSNHLs are controversial for several reasons: there is no definitive cause, not treating could leave a patient with a lifelong disability, and the standard treatment does not have compelling randomized controlled trial data to support it. The American Academy of Otolaryngology-Head and Neck Surgery (AAO-HNS) has established clinical practice guidelines (CPGs) designed to increase diagnostic accuracy, minimize unnecessary tests, provide consistent treatment, and improve outcomes.[10]

HISTORY

Patients with sudden hearing loss typically report symptoms of aural fullness, tinnitus, and possibly vertigo. Individually, these symptoms are not necessarily worrisome and might not raise any concerns on the initial presentation. In fact, it is common for someone with a cerumen impaction or an effusion to have decreased hearing; aural fullness; tinnitus; and, on rare occasions, even vertigo. Therefore, it is important to rule out any history of head trauma, recent ear infections, fevers, or systemic illness. Patients with an ISSNHL will commonly describe waking up with no hearing in 1 ear or perceiving sounds as very distorted like a blown speaker.[9] They will also report that these symptoms came on abruptly and have been persistent since onset. However, patients are unable to describe their symptoms to a degree that allows differentiation of a conductive hearing loss (CHL) from a sensorineural hearing loss, so physical examination skills are key to differentiating between the 2 categories of hearing loss in the primary care setting.

In the case previously described, the patient has no other health issues. He has no history of working in noisy environments, no recent noise exposure, and he specifically denies use of firearms. He denies any trauma, ear drainage, ear pain, or fever. He has never needed chronic medications and is not currently taking any medications or supplements. He denies any other neurologic changes.

PHYSICAL EXAMINATION

The first recommendation from the AAO-HNS CPGs panel is to distinguish a sensori-neural hearing loss from a CHL.[10] By way of review of hearing physiology: the auditory system can be conveniently divided up into 4 sections. The outer and middle ear forms the conductive mechanism, which is responsible for gathering and amplifying incoming sound. The inner ear is the sensory mechanism and is responsible for encod-ing sound into signals that the brain can understand. These encoded signals are routed to the brain along the eighth cranial nerve, which forms the neural mechanism. Finally, the brain processes all of this information and makes sense of the perceived sound. As the name implies, an SSNHL affects the sensory and/or neural mecha-nisms, whereas a disorder such as otitis media with effusion affects the performance of the conductive mechanism. Although the presenting symptoms may be quite similar, the treatment of each is likely to be very different.

A thorough ear examination must be performed with visualization of the tympanic membrane (TM) and evaluation of movement of the TM with pneumatic insufflation. If the TM cannot be visualized, an attempt should be made to clear the canal for full visualization. Even with visualization of the TM, there is poor reliability in diagnosing middle ear effusions between providers.[11] Beyond direct visualization, the most defin-itive ways to determine the location of the hearing disruption is through tympanometry and comprehensive audiometry. These tests are typically performed by an audiologist; however, these services may not be available at the time the patient presents with the symptoms, and a delay in treatment may significantly affect the outcome.

TUNING FORK TESTING

Through the use of an inexpensive and readily available low-frequency tuning fork (256 or 512 Hz), the clinician can differentiate between disorders of the conductive mech-anism (eg, otitis media with effusion) and sensory and/or neural disorders, such as an SSNHL.[12] Tuning fork tests will compare hearing function between the 2 ears, helping to determine if an asymmetry of hearing exists, and whether the pathologic condition in the affected ear is in the conductive or the sensory and/or neural mechanism.[13]

A tuning fork can deliver sound to a patient in 2 different ways. One way is air con-duction, in which the sound is presented to the patient by means of an air medium. The second is bone conduction, in which the sound of the tuning fork is conducted more directly to the inner ear by vibration through bone. For bone conduction, the stem of the tuning fork needs to be in contact with the skull. Because the cochlea is encased in the temporal bone of the skull, these bony vibrations can directly stimulate the sensory organ of hearing.

Weber Test

The 2 most essential tuning fork tests, the Weber and the Rinne, can help determine if a hearing loss is conductive or sensorineural,[10] which will ultimately assist the clinician in the management of the hearing disorder. The Weber tuning fork test uses the bone conduction pathway to send the sound to both ears. The tuning fork is struck into vi-bration, and the stem is placed onto the midline of the skull at the forehead. The pa-tient is then asked where they perceive the sound. If the patient does not hear the tone or is uncertain, the bridge of the nose or maxillary teeth (with gauze covering) may be used for tuning fork placement. The typical responses include the perception of sound in the center of the head (indicating symmetric hearing) or the lateralization of the sound to 1 side or the other, which is documented as Weber lateralized to the left side. For example, in cases in which the disorder is within the conductive mechanism, the sound will lateralize to the ear affected by the conductive disorder. In cases in which the disorder is in the sensory and/or neural mechanism, the sound will lateralize to better ear.[14]

Rinne Test

The Rinne tuning fork test uses both the bone-conduction pathway and the air-conduction pathway. The tuning fork is set into vibration and tines are placed near the patient's external auditory meatus. The stem of the tuning fork is then placed on the mastoid, and the patient is asked to compare the loudness of each placement.[15] If the air-conducted (AC) sound is perceived as being louder than the bone-conducted (BC) sound, then the test is considered positive (AC>BC). This suggests that there is little or no conductive component to the hearing loss. If the BC sound is perceived as being louder than the AC sound, then the test is considered negative (BC > AC). In this case, the loss is considered to have a conductive component.[13] In the case of an SSNHL, the Weber tuning fork test would lateralize away from the affected ear, to the stronger ear. The Rinne test should be either positive (AC > BC) on the ear of concern if the loss is not conductive or not perceived at all by the affected ear if the hearing loss is total.

Tuning fork tests can be very useful in differentiating conductive loss versus sensorineural loss. However, they can sometimes be difficult to interpret and, at times, could be misleading.[16,17] The classic pathways for CHLs and SNHLs are shown in **Fig. 1**. A critical assumption of tuning fork testing is normal baseline hearing. Without this condition being met, it is difficult to interpret the findings.

HUM TEST

If a clinician does not have access to tuning forks and still needs to try to make a determination between a conductive hearing loss and an SNHL, a hum test may be used.[18] The hum test is performed by having the patient hum at a low frequency and report if the hum is louder in 1 ear or the other.[9] This test roughly approximates the Weber test by using bone conduction of the patient-produced sound to their inner ears. As such, with an SNHL, the hum would be diminished in the affected ear and louder in the opposite ear. Conversely, conductive loss would be louder in the affected ear. As a reminder of the lateralization of a CHL, plug 1 ear with a fingertip and hum. This canal occlusion will mimic a CHL.[9]

The remainder of the physical examination should be focused primarily on neurologic function. Any focal neurologic findings should raise concern for a central disease process and consideration for immediate referral.

LABORATORY TESTING

Routine laboratory tests and imaging should not be obtained in patients with a suspected ISSNHL at their initial presentation.[10] The clinical guidelines specifically reference this to avoid a knee-jerk response of ordering a battery of laboratory tests. Endemic issues or suspicion of other underlying causes may prompt focused diagnostic studies and, after the patient has had a formal workup with audiology and otolaryngology evaluations, further studies are likely.

To return to the case study, it is suspected that this patient has an ISSNHL in the right ear. If this assumption is correct, the provider would expect the Weber tuning fork to lateralize to his left ear because inner ear function is diminished on the right. The Rinne test would be positive on both sides, with air conduction exceeding bone conduction.

WEBER TEST   RINNE TEST

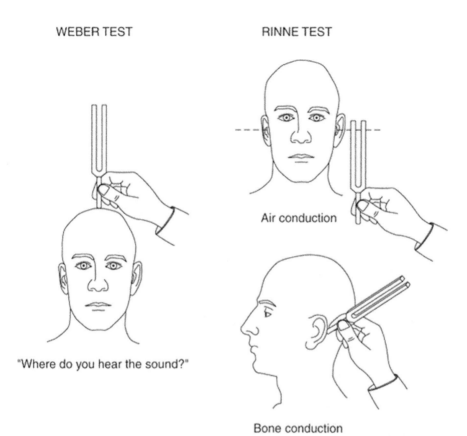

Air conduction

"Where do you hear the sound?"

Bone conduction

Fig. 1. Weber and Rinne tuning fork tests. In the Weber test (*left*), the clinician holds the vibrating tuning fork in the midline against the patient's vertex, forehead, or bridge of nose and asks, "Where do you hear the sound?" In the Rinne test (*right*), the clinician tests 1 ear at a time, comparing perception of sound conducted through air (top right) to perception of sound conducted through bone (bottom right). When testing air conduction, the tuning fork is held so that an axis through both external auditory canals (*dashed line*) passes through both tines of the fork. When testing bone conduction, the stem of the vibrating fork is held against the mastoid. (*From* McGee S. Hearing. In: McGee S. Evidence-based physical diagnosis. 2nd edition. Philadelphia: Elsevier; 2007; with permission.)

TREATMENT: URGENT

Once an ISSNHL is suspected, the ideal next step is an urgent referral to otolaryngology; however, approximately 20% of primary care practices are located outside of areas with otolaryngology services.[7] Even when otolaryngology consultation is available within the community, an urgent referral may not be possible, therefore the current recommendation is to initiate treatment with oral steroids at the time of diagnosis. Waiting for an audiogram or specialty consultation should not delay treatment,[18] which should proceed based on history, physical examination, and tuning fork testing.[19] A classic study by Byl[4] shows a much greater response to treatment at 0 to 7 days. A 2017 study shows earlier treatment seems better but is not significant until 21 days.[20] The consensus throughout the literature is that earlier intervention leads to a better prognosis, so prompt treatment is recommended. However, there is no consensus regarding an endpoint beyond which no treatment is warranted. Treat immediately once identified.

ORAL STEROID THERAPY

Oral corticosteroids are the most widely used therapeutic intervention for an ISSNHL[19] on initial presentation and the most appropriate treatment option in the primary care setting. Oral prednisone is the most commonly cited treatment and is started at a single dose of 1 mg/kg/d up to 60 mg daily with a total duration of 10 to 14 days.[10] Other corticosteroids can be selected, but adjustment must be made to maintain adequate dosing. Relative to hydrocortisone, prednisone is 4 times, methylprednisolone 5 times, and dexamethasone 25 times stronger. So, the typical equivalents to 60 mg of prednisone are 48 mg methylprednisolone or 10 mg of dexamethasone.[10] A typical methylprednisolone dose pack is not sufficient to treat an ISSNHL.

Treatment of ISSNHLs is controversial and clinical judgment is necessary. The use of corticosteroids is not without side effects and should be discussed with patients. The most common side effects include insomnia, dizziness, weight gain, increased sweating, gastritis, mood changes, photosensitivity, and hyperglycemia.[10] Consideration of these side effects; previous patient tolerance to corticosteroids; and other systemic issues, such as poorly controlled diabetes, hypertension, and history of gastric ulcers, should help guide the decision to treat. Multiple previous studies, a Cochrane review, and additional meta-analyses have suggested improvement but not with statistical significance.[19] Up to two-thirds of cases will have some spontaneous recovery of hearing, but the possibility of avoiding potentially permanent hearing loss makes a compelling case in favor of treatment.

To return to the case study patient, there is a high suspicion for an ISSNHL based on his history and the tuning fork examinations. He does not have diabetes, hypertension, peptic ulcer disease, or previous difficulties with corticosteroids. A discussion of risks and potential side-effects has occurred. This patient is concerned about what is going to happen next, and he wonders what other options exist should the oral steroids not prove beneficial.

REFERRAL FOR SPECIALTY CARE

Once treatment has been initiated, a referral to otolaryngology is still recommended. It is important to establish a baseline hearing level to measure effectiveness of treatment. An audiogram will be done to confirm level of hearing loss (**Figs. 2–4**), type of hearing loss (sensorineural and/or conductive), and word recognition. The otolaryngologist will examine the patient once again and correlate the history, physical examination, and audiological findings. If the diagnosis remains an ISSNHL, an MRI will likely be ordered because there is up to a 10% incidence of cerebellopontine angle tumors in patients diagnosed with an SNHL.[10]

INTRATYMPANIC STEROID THERAPY

Patients will be followed closely by otolaryngology providers during their treatment course to monitor for improvement. Other treatment options have shown some potential benefit above and beyond the initial course of oral steroids. One such therapy is intratympanic steroid injection, which can be used as a salvage therapy or as an initial therapy. Another potential therapy, considered optional in the CPGs by AAO-HNS, is hyperbaric oxygen therapy, but there are very little data to support this currently and there is a high financial burden.

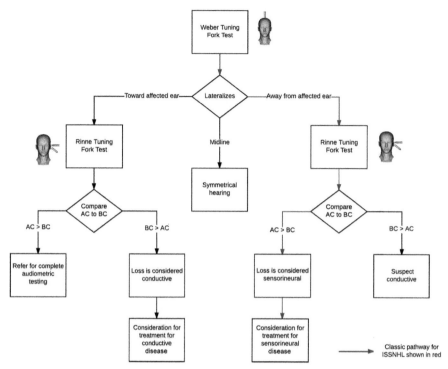

Fig. 2. The classic pathways for CHLs and SNHLs.

Intratympanic steroid therapy can be used as a primary treatment or a salvage treatment. Patients with contraindications to oral steroids are more likely able to tolerate intratympanic steroids as an alternative initial therapy. Like oral steroids, data have been inconsistent regarding efficacy. Some early studies, although small, have shown a significant effect in 14 of 16 subjects.[21] Intratympanic steroids are generally placed via a small gauge needle through an anesthetized portion of the TM over a series of days or intermittently over several weeks. After an injection, the patient remains in the office for up to 30 minutes, lying in a lateral decubitus position, with the affected ear up, facilitating the high-dose steroid solution remaining in the middle ear. The steroid crosses the round window into the inner ear, creating a higher steroid concentration in the perilymph.

Intratympanic regimens vary widely. Frequencies range from 7 to 10 days between applications to multiple instillations per day for patients after a pressure equalization tube is placed.[10] The most common intratympanic steroids used are dexamethasone, 10 mg/mL to 24 mg/mL, and solumedrol, typically at concentrations 30 mg/mL and higher. The variability in treatment regimens and formulations of steroids used has made it difficult to study the effects of intratympanic steroid therapy. Although enacting this treatment is outside the scope of a primary care provider, it is important to discuss these options with the patient, especially beyond the initial 2-week window.

Often, the mention of intratympanic steroids elicits a negative response from patients, due to concerns about procedural risks and discomfort. Although intratympanic steroid therapies are generally safe and well-tolerated, it is important to discuss the risks of pain, dizziness, infection, chronic TM perforation, and vasovagal or syncopal episodes, as well as the cost of treatment and repeated visits.[10] Contextualizing the

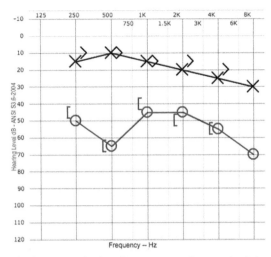

Fig. 3. Audiometric findings. Standard audiometry reveals a graph of the relationship of the patient's hearing level across a range of frequencies. The vertical axis shows the patient's hearing level in decibels (dB). Lower numbers represent little or no hearing loss, although higher numbers represent more significant hearing loss. The horizontal axis indicates the frequency, in hertz (Hz), of the test stimulus. The symbols on the audiogram indicate how the tone was presented to the patient and the softest level (threshold) that they can hear. The blue Xs and the red Os show the thresholds for the left ear and right ear presented through headphones. The brackets (> and [) indicate that the sound was presented to the patient using bone conduction. This method essentially bypasses the outer and middle ears and stimulates the inner ear directly. This audiogram shows that the patient has normal hearing sensitivity in the left ear (blue Xs) and that there is no difference in how they hear by air conduction compared with bone conduction in that ear. Testing of the right ear indicates that there is significant hearing loss at all frequencies. Because the bone-conduction symbols ([) for the right ear show similar thresholds, the hearing loss is considered sensorineural in nature.

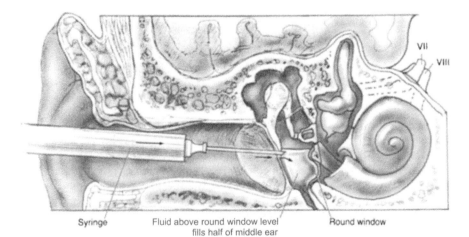

Syringe   Fluid above round window level   Round window
                 fills half of middle ear

Fig. 4. Intratympanic injection of corticosteroid through a pinhole perforation. Corticosteroid is instilled to fill the middle ear ensuring coverage of the round window for diffusion into the inner ear. (*From* Monsell EM, Cass SP, Rybak LP, et al. Chemical treatment of the labyrinth. In: Brackmann DE, Shelton C, Arriaga MA, editors. Otologic surgery, 3rd edition. Philadelphia: Elsevier; 2010; with permission.)

temporary nature of these possible side effects with the opportunity to prevent a life-long hearing deficit, most patients consider intratympanic steroid therapy to be a desirable treatment option, particularly patients with contraindications to systemic oral steroids, those who have failed oral steroid therapy, or those who present more than 1 to 4 weeks from onset of hearing loss.

Prognosis

The longstanding consensus has been that the best chance of recovery from an ISSNHL occurs when a patient is evaluated and treated within 7 days.[4] Most optimistic estimates are that 50% to 70% of patients will recover fully,[4,20] whereas the remainder generally have poor recovery or may worsen. These results are irrespective of type of intervention or lack of treatment. Prognosis seems to mostly depend on the severity of hearing loss at presentation, age, associated vertigo, and time from onset to treatment. Mild hearing loss will typically recover fully without treatment, but severe to profound loss is unlikely to recover fully.[10] Increasing age is a negative predictor for full recovery. One 2015 study of intratympanic steroids found that the probability of a 22-year-old patient having therapeutic success was 60%, whereas a 65-year-old patient's likelihood of improvement was 40%.[22] The presence of tinnitus was found to be a statistically significant positive predictor in a 2017 retrospective study on hearing outcomes with an ISSNHL.[20]

SUMMARY

The goal of the provider caring for a patient with an ISSNHL is to prevent further hearing loss, recover existing hearing loss, and reassure the patient when possible. The AAO-HNS CPGs also outline interventions that should be avoided to minimize financial burden: unnecessary medications and unnecessary studies. In addition to routine laboratory assessment, it is recommended to avoid routine computed tomography scans and pharmacologic therapy outside of corticosteroids, such as antivirals, thrombolytics, vasodilators, vasoactive substances, or antioxidants[10] because none of these treatments have shown benefit outweighing the likelihood of harm.

To return to the 56-year-old patient who presented for care on a Friday afternoon at 4:30 PM noting decreased hearing over the prior 24 hours: the provider must allow sufficient pause for thought. The clinician should take into consideration that sudden hearing loss can be the result of a significant underlying disease process, and that failure to recognize and treat this condition appropriately may lead to lifelong hearing loss that might have otherwise have been avoided.

REFERENCES

1. Alexander TH, Harris JP. Incidence of sudden sensorineural hearing loss. Otol Neurotol 2013;34(9):1586–9.
2. Klemm E, Deutscher A, Mösges R. A present investigation of the epidemiology in idiopathic sudden sensorineural hearing loss. Laryngorhinootologie 2009;88(8): 524–7 [in German].
3. Conlin AE, Parnes LS. Treatment of sudden sensorineural hearing loss: I. A systematic review. Arch Otolaryngol Head Neck Surg 2007;133(6):573–81.
4. Byl FM. Sudden hearing loss: eight years' experience and suggested prognostic table. Laryngoscope 1984;94(5):647.
5. Nosrati-Zarenoe R, Arlinger S, Hultcrantz E. Idiopathic sudden sensorineural hearing loss: results drawn from the Swedish national database. Acta Otolaryngol 2007;127(11):1168–75.

6. Oh J, Park K, Lee SJ, et al. Bilateral versus unilateral sudden sensorineural hearing loss. Otolaryngol Head Neck Surg 2007;136(1):87–91.
7. Cohen SM, Labadie RF, Haynes DS. Primary care approach to hearing loss: the hidden disability. Ear Nose Throat J 2005;84(1)(26):29–31, 44.
8. National Institute of Deafness and Communication Disorders. Sudden deafness. Sudden deafness. Available at: https://www.nidcd.nih.gov/health/sudden-deafness. Published August 18, 2015. Accessed November 14, 2017.
9. Rauch SD. Idiopathic sudden sensorineural hearing loss. N Engl J Med 2008; 359(8):833–40.
10. Stachler RJ, Chandrasekhar SS, Archer SM, et al. Clinical practice guideline: sudden hearing loss. Otolaryngol Head Neck Surg 2012;146(3_suppl):S1–35.
11. Blomgren K, Pitkäranta A. Is it possible to diagnose acute otitis media accurately in primary health care? Fam Pract 2003;20(5):524–7.
12. Ahmed A, Tsiga-Ahmed F, Hasheem M, et al. Hearing screening techniques for referral purposes: our experience from a rural setting. Ann Trop Med Public Health 2013;6(2):173–8.
13. Vikram KB, Naseeruddin K. Combined tuning fork tests in hearing loss: explorative clinical study of the patterns. J Otolaryngol 2004;33(4):227–34.
14. Asher VA, Kveton JF. Clinical evaluation of hearing loss. In: Hughes GB, Pensak ML, editors. Clinical otology. 2nd edition. New York: Thieme; 1997. p. 159–68.
15. Burkey JM, Lippy WH, Schuring AG, et al. Clinical utility of the 512-Hz Rinne tuning fork test. Am J Otol 1998;19(1):59–62.
16. Burgess LP, Frankel SF, Lepore ML, et al. Tuning fork screening for sudden hearing loss. Mil Med 1988;153(9):456–8.
17. Miltenburg DM. The validity of tuning fork tests in diagnosing hearing loss. J Otolaryngol 1994;23(4):254–9.
18. Leung MA, Flaherty A, Zhang JA, et al. Sudden sensorineural hearing loss: primary care update. Hawaii J Med Public Health 2016;75(6):172–4.
19. Lawrence R, Thevasagayam R. Controversies in the management of sudden sensorineural hearing loss: an evidence-based review. Clin Otolaryngol 2015; 40(3):176–82.
20. Ganesan P, Kothandaraman PP, Swapna S, et al. A retrospective study of the clinical characteristics and post-treatment hearing outcome in idiopathic sudden sensorineural hearing loss. Audiol Res 2017;7(1):10–4.
21. Battaglia A, Burchette R, Cueva R. Combination therapy (intratympanic dexamethasone + high-dose prednisone taper) for the treatment of idiopathic sudden sensorineural hearing loss. Otol Neurotol 2008;29(4):453–60.
22. Attanasio G, Covelli E, Cagnoni L, et al. Does age influence the success of intratympanic steroid treatment in idiopathic sudden deafness? Acta Otolaryngol 2015;135(10):969–73.

Evaluation and Management of Pediatric Neck Masses
An Otolaryngology Perspective

Denise L. Jackson, PA-C, MA, CCC-SLP

KEYWORDS

- Cervical fascial spaces • Embryology • Congenital • Ectopic tissue
- Vascular malformations • Pediatric neck mass • Lymphadenopathy

KEY POINTS

- A comprehensive knowledge of the borders and contents of the fascial spaces of the neck is essential to the proper evaluation and diagnosis of pediatric neck lesions.
- Cervical neck spaces are characterized as being anterior or posterior triangle, central or lateral, and by level of the neck.
- Most pediatric neck masses can be characterized as congenital, inflammatory, infectious, or neoplastic (benign or malignant).
- The 2 most common congenital neck lesions in children are branchial cleft and thyroglossal duct anomalies.
- Infectious neck masses can be described as acute or chronic, and range in etiology from common viral exanthems to tick-borne illnesses.

INTRODUCTION

Generally, neck masses in children fall into 1 of 3 categories: congenital, inflammatory, or neoplastic. Although malignancies do occur, most neck masses in children are benign in nature. The objective of this article is to provide practitioners guidance in performing comprehensive physical examinations of the pediatric neck mass, clinical decision making and pursuit of pertinent testing, recognizing diagnostic criteria for various entities, and awareness of appropriate treatment plans.

HISTORY

The age of the child at onset and the duration of the mass are both significant diagnostic factors when taking a history. Knowledge of prior or recent infections of the head and

Disclosure Statement: The author has nothing to disclose.
Otolaryngology–Head and Neck Surgery, University of Virginia Medical Center, 1 Hospital Drive, 2nd Floor, OMS, Room 2741, Charlottesville, VA 22903, USA
E-mail address: DJ7Z@hscmail.mcc.virginia.edu

Physician Assist Clin 3 (2018) 245–269
https://doi.org/10.1016/j.cpha.2017.12.003

physicianassistant.theclinics.com

neck is important. History of a known tick bite prompts suspicion for tick-borne illnesses in a child with a neck mass, with the specific illness depending on geographic region of residence. *Bartonella henselae* or toxoplasmosis play an important role in human pathogenicity, and should be considered if there has been exposure to a cat or cat feces. For those with a history of unpasteurized milk product ingestion or contaminated soil exposure, those from endemic regions, those with immunocompromised state, and/or a history of tuberculosis (TB) exposure, etiologic considerations would include atypical mycobacteria, TB, or human immunodeficiency virus (HIV), respectively. A patient history of head or neck radiation should be considered. Family history is also key, because disorders with a clear hereditary pattern such as multiple endocrine neoplasia syndrome type 2, neurofibromatosis, head and neck cancers, autoimmune disorders, or vascular anomalies may be linked to the patient's presenting neck lesion.

PHYSICAL EXAMINATION AND MASS IDENTIFICATION
Mass Location

A comprehensive knowledge of the borders and contents of the fascial spaces of the neck is essential in diagnosing and characterizing pediatric neck lesions.[1] The neck may be divided into central and lateral spaces. The lateral neck is further divided into the anterior triangle and the posterior triangle. Neck lesions are also described according to levels ranging from IA to VI (**Fig. 1**).[2]

The central neck comprises dissection levels IA and VI. Its borders extend midline from the mentum to the sternal notch, with palpable structures including the hyoid bone, thyroid and cricoid cartilage, thyroid gland, and upper trachea.[1] The lateral neck is divided into anterior and posterior triangles, delineated by the sternocleidomastoid (SCM) muscle. The anterior triangle, including neck dissection levels IB to IV, ranges from anterior to

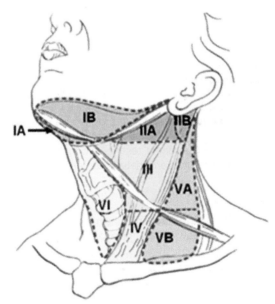

Fig. 1. Neck dissections: radical to conservative. The central neck comprises dissection levels IA (*pink*) and VI (*yellow*). The anterior triangle, including neck dissection levels IB to IV (*pink, purple, green,* and *blue*). From the posterior border of the SCM to thetrapezius muscle and inferiorly to the clavicle (*orange*). (*From* Harish K. Neck dissections: radical to conservative. World J Surg Oncol 2005;3(1):21; with permission.)

the posterior border of the SCM to midline, superiorly along the inferior border of the mandible to the mastoid tip, and inferiorly to the clavicle.[1] The posterior triangle runs from the posterior border of the SCM to the trapezius muscle and inferiorly to the clavicle.[1] Lesions in the supraclavicular fossa have a much higher likelihood of malignancy.[1]

In describing the quality of a neck mass, specific characteristics to include are the size, mobility, tenderness, and appearance of the overlying skin. Benign characteristics include mobility within the soft tissue plane (rather than fixed), well-circumscribed, and small in size. It is important to know if any illness or trauma preceded the mass. Does the lesion fluctuate in size and, if so, what prompts these changes? Drainage or pitting would suggest congenital fistula or deep abscess. If a midline mass elevates with swallowing or tongue protrusion, a thyroglossal duct cyst (TDC) would be likely. In pediatric patients, biopsy is more frequently pursued in larger lesions that persist several weeks, do not resolve with antibiotic therapy, are fixed, or are in the supraclavicular fossa.

Comprehensive Head and Neck Examination

In addition to describing mass location and quality, a complete head and neck examination is crucial, including assessments of regional skin, the ears, the nose, and the oral cavity. The skin on the head and neck, including the scalp, is important to assess because insect bites, evidence of trauma, or dermatologic conditions may be identified as the source of lymphadenopathy. Examination of the oral cavity may reveal mucosal or dental lesions that may also contribute to formation of neck masses. Meticulous neck examination, beyond the mass itself, including thyroid inspection and palpation, is fundamental. A gross cranial nerve assessment should also be performed. Flexible nasopharyngolaryngoscopy may be indicated in some cases.

DIAGNOSTIC TESTING
Laboratory Tests

Laboratory tests to consider for the workup of acute lymphadenitis include monospot or serology for Epstein-Barr virus and cytomegalovirus, and/or phlebotomy to include a complete blood count with differential, at a minimum. It is appropriate to culture any material expressed from an abscess or from any surface lesion, that is, a nasaopharyngeal culture for increasingly more common respiratory viruses such as metapneumovirus and respiratory syncytial virus, or tonsillar culture if group A streptococcus is suspected. A *B henselae* immunofluorescence assay blood test assesses for cat scratch disease if there is a history of such an incident or exposure. *Toxoplasma gondii* antibodies (immunoglobulins G and M) should be considered if applicable, as well as Lyme and ehrlichiosis titers, HIV testing, tuberculin skin testing, and a chest radiograph, if the TB test is positive. Acidfast bacilli testing is important in confirming atypical mycobacteria. If thyroid involvement is probable, a thyroid panel may be considered. Further workup largely depends on the location and characteristics of a lesion. If an abscess is present, fine needle aspiration with a Gram stain would be recommended, to facilitate directed antibiotic therapy, along with acid-fast bacilli staining for mycobacteria, if suspected. Flexible nasopharyngolaryngoscopy will often be deemed necessary for upper airway evaluation. If neoplasm is present, laboratory tests and excisional biopsy are confirmatory of diagnosis, and appropriate referrals will need to be made for multidisciplinary management.

Imaging

Various imaging modalities, including ultrasound examination, computed tomography (CT) scans, MRI, and MR angiography are used for the evaluation of pediatric neck lesions, and each has its own advantages, limitations, and indications.[3] The radiologic evaluation of pediatric patients after physical examination often begins with conventional ultrasound examination and color Doppler ultrasound examination owing to its nonionizing and noninvasive ability to depict superficial structures.[3] Ultrasound examination can define the size and extent of localized superficial masses and determine a cystic or solid nature. Color Doppler ultrasound examination can demonstrate the vascularization of the mass, displaced normal surrounding vessels, or intralesional flow.[3] However, ultrasound examination findings may not allow definitive characterization, especially for deeper lesions.[3] CT scanning aids in the morphologic characterization and staging of neck masses, and allows for the precise visualization of fine bone structures, calcifications, and deep soft tissue compartments that cannot be demonstrated with ultrasound examination.[3] Particular attention should be paid to minimizing the radiation exposure of CT scans, particularly in pediatric patients.[3] MRI, with an absence of ionizing radiation and multiplanar capability, offers superior contrast resolution in evaluating masses in complex areas, including the head and neck.[3] CT scanning is a more rapid study than MRI, but either modality may require intravenous sedation for younger patients.[3]

The gold standard for diagnosis of vascular lesions involves MRI with gadolinium and/or Doppler ultrasound examination to measure flow.[4] Arteriovenous malformation and arteriovenous fistula are high-flow lesions, whereas venous and lymphatic malformations are low-flow lesions.[5] Both hemangiomas and vascular anomalies enhance on T2-weighted images.[1] Lymphatic malformations appear as multilocular cystic lesions on ultrasound imaging, and also show hyperintensity on T2-weighted MRI.[4] For embryologic tracts, MRI with fistulogram helps to determine the extent and final disposition of the tract. Each case warrants careful consideration regarding imaging so as to obtain the greatest yield with the least risk to the patient.

EMBRYOLOGY
Branchial Apparatus

A comprehensive review of head and neck embryology is beyond the scope of this article. However, a brief review of the embryologic pathway for the branchial apparatus, which is determined in the first 8 weeks in utero, informs our understanding of congenital neck masses.[6] The branchial apparatus consists of paired pharyngeal arches, pharyngeal pouches, pharyngeal clefts (or grooves), and pharyngeal membranes.[6] Pharyngeal arches are paired structures that contribute to the formation of the face, jaw, ear, and neck.[6] The first pharyngeal arch appears around the beginning of the fourth week and others are sequentially added more caudally, with 5 arches present by the end of the fourth gestational week; the fifth arch halts in development, such that the remaining arches are numbered 1, 2, 3, 4, and 6.[6] The pharyngeal apparatus forms infoldings or pouches between the arches.[6] Externally, the pharyngeal apparatus forms outer pharyngeal clefts (or grooves).[6] Anomalies of the branchial apparatus can present as fistulas (incomplete closure of pouches and clefts, resulting in communication between 2 body surfaces), cysts (trapped embryologic remnants with no external communication), and sinuses (incomplete closure of pouches and clefts, with single body surface communication involving skin or pharynx).[1] Specific types of branchial apparatus anomalies are highlighted elsewhere in the article.

CONGENITAL NECK MASSES
Central Congenital Neck Masses

Thyroglossal duct cysts
TDCs are the most common congenital neck masses. They are midline lesions that arise as the result of a residual tract left by the thyroid gland during its embryologic

descent from the foramen cecum at the base of the tongue, downward to its definitive position[1] (**Figs. 2–4**). TDCs characteristically elevate with tongue protrusion or swallowing.[1] They are very well-circumscribed, mobile, and nontender. Often, TDCs go unrecognized until they enlarge in response to an infection; therefore, the most common age of presentation is in young, school-aged children.[1] MRI or CT scans can delineate the full extent of the lesion for perioperative planning; however, ultrasound imaging may be sufficient for radiologic assessment of a central neck mass with a high suspicion for TDC.[1] Confirmation of normally functional thyroid tissue before TDC resection is also accomplished through preoperative imaging. Once confirmed, a Sistrunk procedure is typically performed, which involves surgical resection of the cystic lesion, along with the entire tract of embryologic descent, up to and including the tract insertion onto a portion of the hyoid bone, thus drastically reducing the rate of TDC recurrence.[1] This type of surgical intervention is curative in the majority of patients.

Dermoid and epidermoid cysts

In contrast with TDCs, dermoid and epidermoid cysts are midline lesions (**Fig. 5**), which do not typically elevate with swallowing or tongue protrusion. Like TDCs, dermoid and epidermoid cysts are characteristically well-circumscribed and typically nontender. These cysts are extremely mobile, and superficial to underlying structures. Dermoid cysts are lined by epithelium and differ from epidermoid cysts in that they contain skin appendages such as sebaceous glands and hair follicles within the cyst wall.[4] Dermoids may present in later childhood owing to their slow evolution. Forty percent of dermoid and epidermoid cysts are diagnosed at birth, with the majority of the remaining 60% of these cysts presenting before the age of 5 years.[1] On noncontrast CT, a dermoid cyst usually appears as a low-density, unilocular,

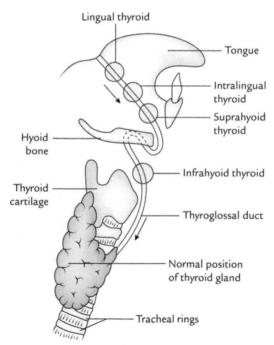

Fig. 2. Path of thyroglossal duct. Note the possible locations of thyroid tissue and thyroglossal cysts in this path. (*From* Coward K, Wells D, editors. Textbook of clinical embryology. Philadelphia: Elsevier; 2012. p. 122–9; with permission.)

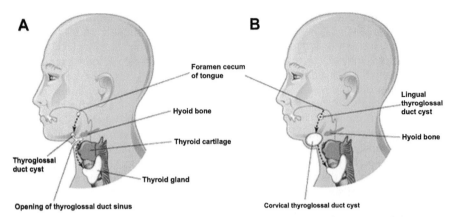

Fig. 3. Arteriovenous malformation of the lower lip. (*A*) Opening of thyroglossal duct sinus. (*B*) Cervical thyroglossal duct cyst. (*From* Coward K, Wells D, editors. Textbook of clinical embryology. Philadelphia: Elsevier; 2012. p. 122–9; with permission.)

well-circumscribed mass.[4] Fat, mixed-density fluid, and calcification (<50%) may also be seen, and there may be coalescence of fat into small nodules within the cystic lesion, giving a "sack of marbles" appearance (**Fig. 6**).[4] The presence of calcifications and cystic spaces in these lesions aids in their differentiation from lipomas.[4] Patients respond well to surgical excision, which is typically curative.

Plunging ranula

Plunging ranulas may be either congenital or acquired lesions. Their pathophysiology involves obstruction of a sublingual gland, which forms a pseudocyst or mucocele along the floor of the mouth. This cyst becomes termed a "plunging ranula" when the lesion extends into the neck through the mylohyoid[1] (**Fig. 7**). Preoperative imaging

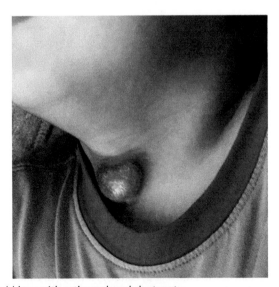

Fig. 4. A 4-year-old boy with a thyroglossal duct cyst.

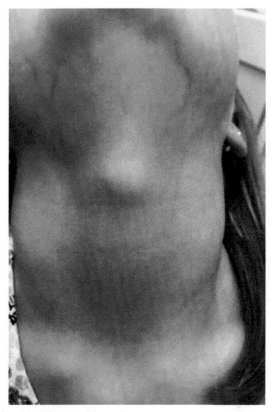

Fig. 5. A 5-year-old girl with an epidermal cyst.

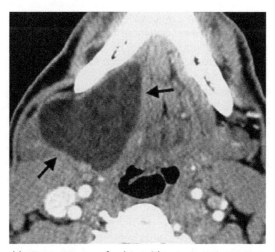

Fig. 6. "Sack of marbles" appearance of a dermoid cyst, as seen on a computed tomography scan (*arrows*). (*From* Friedman ER, John SD. Imaging of pediatric neck masses. Radiol Clin North Am 2011. https://doi.org/10.1016/j.rcl.2011.05.005; 49(4):617–32; with permission.)

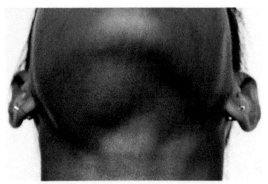

Fig. 7. Plunging ranula. (*From* Mahadevan M, Vasan N. Management of pediatric plunging ranula. Int J Pediatr Otorhinolaryngol 2006;70(6):1049–54; with permission.)

is paramount to ensuring complete excision and avoiding injury to the surrounding structures.

Midline cervical clefts

Midline congenital anomalies are congenital neck lesions that result from impaired fusion of branchial arches in the anterior neck are called midline cervical clefts.[7] They can extend from mandible to manubrium, presenting as a linear vertical area of thin and erythematous mucosa at birth.[7] There is often a projection from the upper portion of the lesion and a sinus or fistula inferiorly.[7] Sometimes, there is a fibrous band beneath the mucosal defect, as well[7] (**Fig. 8**). If not treated early, the midline cord begins to tether the anterior neck as the infant grows.[7] Thus, surgical excision has both cosmetic and functional benefits.

LATERAL CONGENITAL NECK MASSES
Branchial Cleft Anomalies

Branchial arches form the embryologic precursors of the ear, as well as the muscles, vasculature, bones, cartilage, and mucosal lining of the face, neck, and pharynx.[8] Branchial arch anomalies are the second most common head and neck congenital lesions in children and represent approximately 20% of cervical masses in the pediatric population.[8] Second branchial arch anomalies are the most common and account for approximately 95% of cases.[8]

Branchial cleft anomalies arise from incomplete obliteration of any branchial tract, resulting in a cyst, a sinus, or a fistula. Branchial cleft cysts are fluid filled, and the material expressed from them may resemble brown motor oil. They are commonly well-circumscribed, painless, and mobile. Branchial cleft cysts have no external opening. Branchial cleft sinus tracts occur from incomplete closure of clefts and pouches, yet have single body surface communication, either to pharynx or skin.[1] Branchial cleft fistulas form similarly, but communicate with 2 body surfaces.[1] Cysts more commonly present in older children, whereas fistulas are more often recognized in infancy or younger children.[8]

First Branchial Cleft Anomalies

First branchial cleft cysts are the most cephalad of the anomalies. They are rare (<1%), typically originate from the angle of the mandible, extend to the external auditory canal, and are often associated with the facial nerve.[1] First branchial cleft

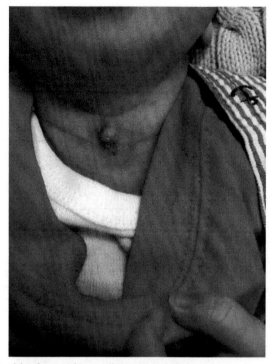

Fig. 8. A 3-month-old infant with a midline cervical cleft.

cysts are further characterized as either Work type I (preauricular, extending to ear canal or middle ear) or Work type II (angle of mandible, extending to concha or ear canal).[1]

Second Branchial Cleft Anomalies

Second branchial cleft anomalies are the most common (95%) of the 4 types, with cysts occurring more frequently than sinuses or fistulas.[1] Unilateral and right-sided presentations are most common.[1] Second branchial cleft anomalies are located in close proximity to the internal jugular vein.[7] Fistulas open to the skin along the anterior border of the SCM muscle, dive deep between second and third branchial arch structures to course between the external and internal carotid arteries, lateral to glossopharyngeal and hypoglossal nerves, medial to posterior belly of the digastric and stylohyoid, and ultimately connect to the tonsillar fossa.[1] Second branchial cleft anomalies can be associated with branchiootorenal syndrome, so auditory and renal screening is important upon diagnosis of this particular congenital neck lesion.[1]

Third and Fourth Branchial Cleft Anomalies

Like first branchial cleft anomalies, third and fourth branchial cleft cysts are rarely encountered. They are typically located lower in the neck than second branchial cleft cysts, along the inferior-most one-third of the anterior border of the SCM muscle. Sinus tracts, if present, ascend along the carotid sheath posteriorly toward the internal carotid artery, under the glossopharyngeal nerve, and over the vagus and hypoglossal nerves, to open into the piriform sinus or thyrohyoid membrane.

Third and fourth branchial cleft anomalies are distinguished anatomically by their relationship to the superior laryngeal nerve with third pharyngeal cleft anomalies above the nerve, and fourth pharyngeal cleft anomalies below.[8] Most third branchial cleft cysts present in the posterior cervical space (posterior to the SCM muscle) as painless, fluctuant masses that may enlarge and become tender if infected.[8] An infected third branchial cleft cyst should be considered when a pediatric patient presents with an abscess in the posterior triangle of the neck.[8]

A fourth branchial cleft fistula or sinus tract arises from the pyriform sinus apex and descends inferiorly into the mediastinum along the path of the tracheoesophageal groove.[8] These branchial cleft anomalies are commonly left sided and most often present as a sinus tract coursing from the apex of the pyriform fossa to the upper aspect of the left thyroid lobe.[8]

Management of Branchial Cleft Anomalies

Surgical excision is curative and a commonly chosen option for treatment of branchial cleft anomalies, particularly if there is recurrent infection.[8]

Imaging of Branchial Cleft Anomalies

Usually, branchial cleft anomalies are imaged with MRI with contrast (**Fig. 9**). If an overt pit or fistula is evident on examination and amenable to cannulation, then CT neck with fistulogram and 3-dimensional reformatting is preferred (**Fig. 10**).

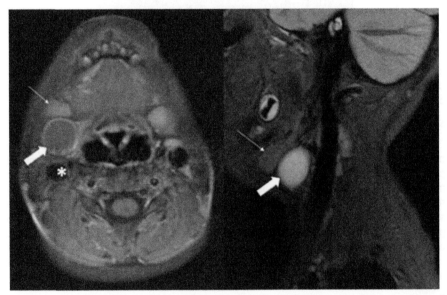

Fig. 9. A 2-year-old child with axial fat-suppressed T1-weighted postcontrast and sagittal short tau inversion recovery images demonstrating a rounded and well-defined T1-weighted isointense, T2-weighted hyperintense lesion with thin peripheral enhancement (*thick white arrows*). This lesion is demonstrated posterior to the right submandibular gland (*thin white arrow*) and anterior to the sternocleidomastoid muscle and carotid sheath (*asterisk*). This diagnosis was confirmed on surgical excision to represent a second branchial cleft cyst. (*From* Adams A, Mankad K, Offiah C, et al. Branchial cleft anomalies: a pictorial review of embryological development and spectrum of imaging findings. Insights Imaging 2016;7(1):69–76; with permission.)

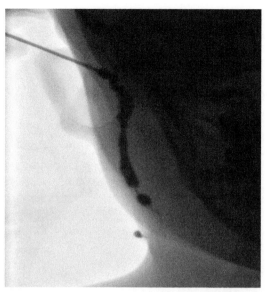

Fig. 10. A sinogram performed on a child before surgical excision of a presumed first bran-chial cleft fistula. The opening within the right external auditory canal was cannulated and water-soluble contrast media was injected, with sinography confirming the presence of a fistulous tract. During the procedure, contrast media was noted to pass via the tract to an external cutaneous opening in the right submandibular region. (*From* Adams A, Mankad K, Offiah C, et al. Branchial cleft anomalies: a pictorial review of embryological development and spectrum of imaging findings. Insights Imaging 2016;7(1):69–76; with permission.)

Torticollis

Torticollis, also known as fibromatosis colli, is an in utero contraction of the SCM mus-cle with fibrous infiltrate, which may present as a neck mass in infancy. The neonate's head is typically tilted laterally toward the ipsilateral affected muscle and the chin is rotated contralateral to the contracture (**Fig. 11**). CT scanning or ultrasound examina-tion shows an isodense oval mass in the SCM muscle.[1] Torticollis can lead to posi-tional plagiocephaly. Physical therapy can help torticollis tremendously. Parents should also be advised to place stimuli on the child's affected side to encourage greater neck range of motion. Imaging and surgical are warranted only if the condition persists beyond the first year of life.

Thymic Cysts

Cervical thymic cysts, like their thyroglossal duct corollary, arise from persistence of the embryologic thymopharyngeal duct, which can occur adjacent to the carotid sheath anywhere from the hyoid bone to the anterior mediastinum.[4] The most common age of presentation of a cervical thymic cyst is 2 to 15 years, with a slight male predilection.[4] Cervical thymic cysts may have a similar appearance to third and fourth branchial cleft cysts, being differentiated only by the presence of thymic tissue upon excision.[4] The cysts usually present as a painless, unilocular cystic mass, extending inferiorly within the neck, paralleling the SCM muscle.[4] They can be found anywhere from the angle of the mandible to the thoracic inlet or mediastinum, more typically on the left side.[9]

Subcategories of cervical thymic lesions include ectopic or undescended thymus (typically not cystic), accessory thymus, cervical thymic cysts, thymopharyngeal

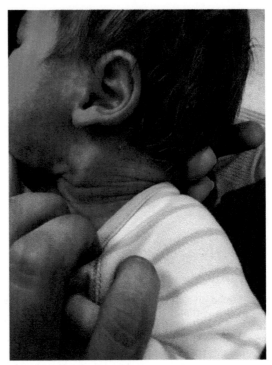

Fig. 11. An 8-week-old infant with a left midsternocleidomastoid mass consistent with congenital torticollis.

duct cyst, and cervical extension of mediastinal thymus (with midline thymus at thoracic inlet).[10] CT scanning or MRI with contrast are standard imaging for diagnosis; the specific study varies by patient and institution. Surgical excision of thymic cysts is typically indicated.

Laryngocele

A laryngocele is formed by a congenital herniation of the saccule of the larynx, and more commonly presents in adulthood rather than the pediatric population.[1] This herniation can be limited to the anatomic boundaries of the larynx (internal laryngocele), or extend through the thyrohyoid membrane (external or mixed laryngocele).[1] When a laryngocele extends beyond the larynx, it often presents as an anterior neck cyst that episodically fills with air.[1] The etiology is suspected to be from a congenital enlargement of the laryngeal saccule, followed by a period of prolonged increased laryngeal pressure (from straining or crying) with a partial obstruction of the neck of the saccule, trapping air within the herniated tissue[1] (**Fig. 12**). An internal laryngocele presents more commonly in infancy as stridor, respiratory distress, feeding problems, and/or chronic cough. In the pediatric population, external laryngocele most commonly presents during the teen years in conjunction with playing a musical instrument that requires increased laryngeal pressure, such as the trumpet. External laryngoceles may form a visible or palpable mass in the neck.[11] Evaluation, particularly with presenting symptoms of airway compromise, may require fiberoptic or direct laryngoscopy. A CT scan with contrast is the most accurate imaging modality for defining spatial relationships between a laryngocele and laryngeal structures, as well as

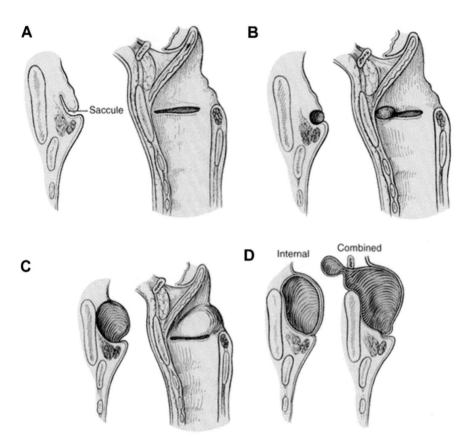

Fig. 12. The classification scheme for a saccular cyst or laryngocele. (*A*) Normal anatomy. (*B*) Anterior saccular cyst. (*C*) Lateral saccular cyst. (*D*) Laryngocele types. Benign vocal fold mucosal disorders. (*From* Richardson M, Flint P, Haughey B, et al. Diagnostic imaging of the pharynx and esophagus. Cummings otolaryngology head & neck surgery. Philadelphia: Elsevier; 2010. https://doi.org/10.1016/B978-0-323-05283-2.00063-X. Fig 62-27; with permission.)

extralaryngeal soft tissues, in differentiating a laryngocele from other cystic formations, and in identifying the coexistence of any laryngeal malignancy[11] (**Fig. 13**). Management, based on severity of symptoms, may include respiratory support with the possible need for intubation and/or tracheostomy, observation, cyst decompression via needle aspiration, endoscopic resection, or resection through an external approach.[11]

CENTRAL AND/OR LATERAL CONGENITAL NECK MASSES
Vascular Anomalies

Vascular lesions of the pediatric neck are typically characterized as either hemangiomas or vascular malformations.[12]

Hemangiomas

Congenital hemangiomas are differentiated from infantile hemangiomas in that congenital hemangiomas are fully formed at birth and do not go through a regression

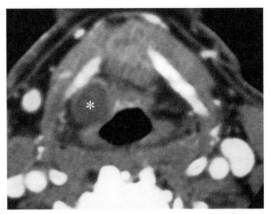

Fig. 13. Intrinsic laryngocele. Enhanced computed tomography of the larynx reveals a fluid-filled mass (*asterisk*) in the paraglottic fat. Laryngoceles may be filled with air or fluid. (*From* Richardson M, Flint P, Haughey B, et al. Diagnostic imaging of the pharynx and esophagus. Cummings otolaryngology head & neck surgery. Philadelphia: Elsevier; 2010. p. 1393–420. Fig 102-18.)

phase.[1] Infantile hemangiomas present soon after birth and undergo proliferation, then involution stages.[1]

Infantile hemangiomas

Infantile hemangiomas may present at birth as flat, violaceous lesions that may be mistaken for a bruise. They become more prominent with crying or straining. They expand by early proliferation and begin to spontaneously involute around 12 months of age, typically never to regrow.[1] The proliferation stage usually starts at 2 to 4 weeks of age, is most rapid in the first 4 to 6 months, and continues through about 1 year of age.[1] Growth of infantile hemangiomas may continue in some cases after a year of age, particularly when involving the airway, when in a beard distribution, or when treated with high-dose steroids.[1] The involution phase starts at about 1 year of age and rate can be extremely variable, ranging from a quick resolution to slow improvement over 10 years.[1]

Congenital hemangiomas

Congenital hemangiomas are fully formed at birth and may be identified on prenatal ultrasound imaging. These lesions are raised, and usually pink to blue color. There are 2 subtypes of congenital hemangiomas: rapidly involuting congenital hemangioma and never involuting congenital hemangioma.[1] Rapidly involuting congenital hemangioma are hemangiomas that are fully developed at birth and immediately begin to involute. Never involuting congenital hemangioma are also fully developed at birth, but maintain their shape and size, and never involute.[13] Involution of rapidly involuting congenital hemangiomas takes place at an estimated rate of 10% per year, so that approximately 50% have involuted by 5 years of age, 70% by 7 years, and 90% by 9 years.[13] An association has been shown between cervicofacial hemangiomas in a beard distribution and subglottic and upper airway hemangiomas; patients with 2 or more hemangiomas along the jawline should be observed for stridor or a crouplike cough. Laryngoscopy is critical at the first sign of stridor or croup in these patients.[14]

PHACES syndrome should be considered in patients with 2 or more of the following for which it is named: posterior fossa abnormalities, hemangioma, arterial abnormalities, cardiac abnormalities, eye abnormalities, and/or sternal cleft or defect.[1] PHACES has been reported in patients with segmental facial hemangiomas as well as in those with isolated, focal hemangiomas[1] (**Fig. 14**). The workup consists of MRI and MR angiography of neck and brain, echocardiogram, and an ophthalmologic assessment.[1]

Diffuse neonatal hemangiomatosis is a rare condition characterized by the presence of numerous cutaneous and visceral hemangiomas that manifest at birth or within the neonatal period. The cutaneous lesions are generalized, vary from 0.5 to 1.5 cm in diameter, and range from 50 to 500 in number. Visceral lesions are most commonly found in the liver, central nervous system, intestine, and lungs. Skeletal involvement has also been reported. Approximately 60% of infants with diffuse neonatal hemangiomatosis die during the first few months of life owing to high-output cardiac failure, hemorrhage, or central nervous system involvement.[1] Steroid therapy is thought to accelerate involution of diffuse neonatal hemangiomatosis lesions.[15]

Management of hemangiomas depends on extent and location of involvement; initially, watchful waiting is often reasonable, because the majority of these lesions resolve spontaneously and the disease process is benign.[1] However, for hemangiomas that are deforming, impair function, or are ulcerated, propranolol (Inderal) has become the first line of therapy with vasoconstriction as the therapeutic objective.[1] This agent should be used in caution in patients with PHACES syndrome.[1] Additional treatment modalities for congenital hemangiomas include topical timolol gel, intralesional steroid injections, chemotherapeutic agents, and laser treatments. Hemangiomas involving the neck and face, although benign, can lead to parental stress, fear, and grief. This factor should be considered when caring for patients with facial hemangioma and their families.

Vascular Malformations

Vascular malformations may or may not be present at birth.[1] These lesions do not involute, but rather will grow with the patient, and so surgical excision is typically required.[12] Several different types of vascular malformations are recognized:

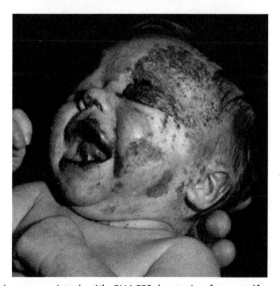

Fig. 14. Hemangioma associated with PHACES (posterior fossa malformations–hemangiomas–arterial anomalies–cardiac defects–eye abnormalities–sternal cleft and supraumbilical raphe) syndrome. (*From* Conlon JD, Drolet BA. Skin lesions in the neonate. Pediatr Clin North Am 2004;51(4):863–88, vii–viii; with permission.)

arteriovenous malformations, venous malformations, capillary malformations, and lymphatic malformations.[1] For vascular anomalies, diagnostic ultrasound can be helpful by determining intraluminal flow and flow voids, but neck MRI with gadolinium and fat suppression, sometimes with MR angiography, is the gold standard.[1] Arteriovenous malformation lesions typically show an infiltrative mass, bright on T1-weighted imaging, along with tissue infiltration and destruction.[1] Both venous and lymphatic malformations exhibit slow flow and enhance on T2-weighted imaging.[1] Ultrasound examination of lymphatic malformations will show a complex, multilocular cystic mass; MRI shows low to intermediate intensity on T1-weighted images, and hyperintensity on T2-weighted images.[1]

Arteriovenous malformations

Arteriovenous malformations are complex masses of arteries and veins associated with rapid blood flow and a high risk of recurrence after treatment.[12] An associated bruit may be present on auscultation. These classically have a superficial blue to bluish-red color and will undergo aggressive growth, resulting in tissue destruction[1] (**Fig. 15**). Embolization is the treatment of choice, for the purpose of limiting growth and control of acute bleeding.[1]

Capillary malformations

Capillary malformations, commonly known as port wine stains, cause light pink to dark red discoloration of the skin.[12] These lesions are typically noted at birth, but differ from

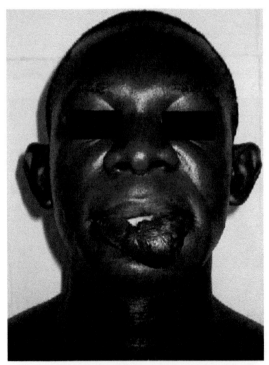

Fig. 15. Arteriovenous malformation of the lower lip. A tobacco-pouch suture technique for the treatment of vascular lesions of the lip in Enugu, Nigeria. (*From* Oji C, Chukwuneke F, Mgbor N. Tobacco-pouch suture technique for the treatment of vascular lesions of the lip in Enugu, Nigeria. Br J Oral Maxillofac Surg 2006;44(3):245–7; with permission.)

hemangiomas in that they do not undergo a proliferative phase.[1] The mainstay of management is serial pulsed dye laser treatment or surgery to treat soft tissue hypertrophy.[1] Facial venous malformations of the forehead, scalp, and eye in V1 and V2 distribution should raise index of suspicion for Sturge-Weber syndrome, also known as encephalotrigeminal angiomatosis, with ocular and central nervous system venous malformations and related impairments.

Venous malformations
Venous malformations are usually deep blue to purple, collapsing with pressure, and swelling with exertion.[1] They can be exacerbated by pregnancy, puberty, menopause, or trauma.[1] Treatment options include laser, sclerotherapy, or surgery.[1]

Lymphatic malformation
Lymphatic malformations (also known as cystic hygroma or lymphangioma) are most commonly found in the posterior cervical triangle of the neck (**Fig. 16**) or submandibular space.[1] These are typically present at birth, at which point approximately 50% are diagnosed, with 90% are identified by the age of 2 years.[1] On physical examination, they have a rubbery, doughlike consistency and do not have well-circumscribed borders, because they do not respect fascial planes. Their violaceous appearance and translumination property distinguish them from other lesions.[1] Lymphatic malformations can be microcystic (capillary lymphangiomas), macrocytic (cavernous

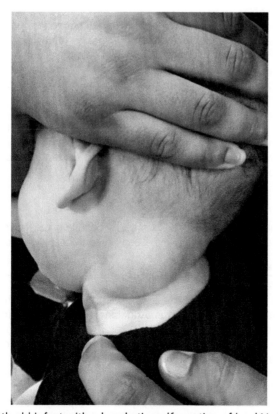

Fig. 16. A 9-month-old infant with a lymphatic malformation of level V of left neck.

lymphangiomas), or mixed. Spontaneous regression occurs in up to 15% of cases for macrocystic lesions.[1] Smaller, asymptomatic macrocystic lymphatic malformations can be observed for up to 24 months.[1] Treatment options for macrocystic lymphangiomas include sclerotherapy with substances such as OK-432 (Picibanil) and/or surgical excision.[1] Microcystic lymphatic malformations are generally not amenable to sclerotherapy and may require serial excision.

Fetal Cervical Lesions

Cervical lesions presenting in the fetal period are often giant in size and may have various etiologies, with cervical lymphangiomas and cervical teratomas being the two most common.

Fetal lymphatic malformations

Lymphatic malformations (described in greater detail elsewhere in this article) may be identified prenatally on fetal ultrasound examination as multiloculated cystic masses that do not respect fascial planes and are not well-circumscribed.[1] Fetal lymphatic malformations that present earlier, during the second trimester, commonly arise from the posterior triangle and have a high rate of association with chromosomal abnormalities (eg, Turner syndrome).[1] With later presentation of fetal lymphangioma (during the third trimester or postnatally), there is less likelihood of an associated chromosomal abnormality, and the location is more commonly within the anterior triangle.[1]

Fetal cervical teratomas

Fetal cervical teratomas of the head and neck are uncommon, comprising less than 5% of all teratomas.[1] They may be found in the second trimester on fetal ultrasound examination and typically present as a rapidly enlarging lateral or midline neck mass, which frequently causes airway obstruction.[1] Teratomas have more defined borders than lymphangiomas and a more heterogenous appearance.[1] They are associated with maternal polyhydramnios in 30% of cases.[1]

Management of these very large fetal neck masses involves a multidisciplinary, carefully planned surgical birth via ex utero intrapartum treatment (EXIT procedure) to deliver the head and neck, secure the neonate's airway with tracheostomy, then complete the delivery.[1] Complete excision of the cervical teratoma or lymphangioma can then be performed[1] (**Fig. 17**).

INFECTIOUS AND INFLAMMATORY NECK MASSES

Acute inflammatory or infections neck masses, by definition, are those present for less than 2 weeks, and chronic masses have been present for 2 weeks or more.[1]

Acute Infectious and Inflammatory Neck Masses

Cervical lymphadenitis

Two of the most common viral causes of pediatric cervical lymphadenopathy are Epstein–Barr virus and cytomegalovirus. Additional culprits include influenza, parainfluenza, rhinovirus, adenovirus, and coronavirus. Pediatric viral exanthems such as mumps, measles, and coxsackie viruses can also cause cervical lymphadenopathy. Bacterial etiologies include *Streptococcus pyogenes* and *Staphylococcus aureus*, although methicillin-resistant *S aureus* is increasing. Sources of infection resulting in cervical lymphadenopathy include otitis media, adenoiditis, tonsillitis, and skin and scalp lesions. Infectious and inflammatory lymphadenopathy is usually tender. There are often associated constitutional symptoms, including malaise and fever. If

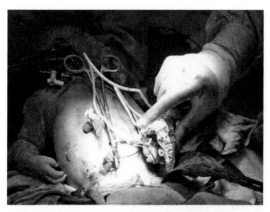

Fig. 17. Ex utero intrapartum treatment procedure. (*From* Marwan A, Crombleholme T. The EXIT procedure: principles, pitfalls, and progress. Semin Pediatr Surg 2006;15(2):107–15; with permission.)

resolution of lymphadenopathy occurs with use of antibiotic therapy, no further laboratory tests or imaging studies are typically required. When lymphadenopathy is unresponsive to oral antibiotics, observation, incision and drainage, pertinent laboratory tests, and/or imaging studies may be warranted.

Chronic Infectious and Inflammatory Neck Masses

Atypical mycobacterial infection

Atypical mycobacterial infection presents in the pediatric neck as a painless, fluctuant lymph node with a violaceous appearance of the overlying skin, and eventual breakdown of skin with necrosis[1] (**Fig. 18**). This organism is found in dirt or unpasteurized milk products.[1] Infected individuals typically have a positive PPD test result.[1] Treatment includes antibiotic therapy, typically a macrolide, in conjunction with an antimycobacterial agent such as rifampin (Rafidan) for 12 weeks at minimum. Surgical excision is ultimately necessary and pathology classically shows necrotizing granulomatous inflammation, staining positive for acid-fast bacilli.

Toxoplasmosis

Toxoplasmosis is a disease caused by a very common parasite, *Toxoplasma gondii*.[1] Infection with this parasite can be acquired by changing cat litter boxes, consuming undercooked meats (from an infected animal), through blood transfusion, or via placental transmission.[1] Infected children may be asymptomatic or can present with flulike symptoms and cervical lymphadenitis. A diagnosis of toxoplasmosis is made via antibody testing, with elevated levels of immunoglobulin M (earlier disease) and immunoglobulin G (later disease).[1] The condition is typically self-limited unless the patient is immunocompromised.[1]

Bartonella

Cat scratch disease can develop over weeks to months in children who have had exposure to cats, with or without a recalled history of a cat scratch.[1] Serologic testing for *B henselae* is positive in infected individuals, who present with a painless and fluctuant cervical mass. The condition is self-limited, although treatment with antibiotics may be recommended, particularly for immunocompromised children.[1]

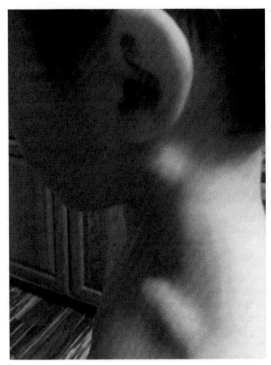

Fig. 18. A 6-year-old child with an atypical mycobacteria infection.

Human immunodeficiency virus

HIV infection commonly causes generalized lymphadenopathy, often involving the cervical and occipital nodes.[1] Identification obtained via HIV serology and treatment is per infectious disease protocol.

Tick-Borne Illnesses

Lyme disease

Lyme disease, the most common vector-borne infection in the United States, is caused by the spirochete *Borrelia burgdorferi*.[16] The majority of cases occur in the Northeastern coastal regions, the upper Midwest, and northern California.[16] Early localized disease is characterized by erythema migrans, classically an erythematous and enlarging "bulls eye" rash.[16] Mild systemic complaints, such as fever, fatigue, myalgias, arthralgias, headache, and cervical lymphadenopathy, may accompany erythema migrans.[16] Positive Lyme antibody screening tests should be confirmed by Western blot test.[16] Doxycycline (Vibramycin) is recommended for treatment of early localized and early disseminated disease, whereas ceftriaxone (Rocephin) is preferred for Lyme meningitis and late disseminated disease.[16]

Ehrlichiosis and Rocky Mountain Spotted Fever

Other tick-borne illnesses may present similarly with symptoms including, but not limited to, lymphadenopathy, fatigue, fever, rash, and myalgias.[16] *Ehrlichia chaffeensis* is the agent responsible for human monocytic ehrlichiosis. Most reported cases of human monocytic ehrlichiosis infection occur in the South and Southeast, and *Amblyomma americanum* and *Dermacentor variabilis* are the principal tick vectors.[16] *Rickettsia rickettsia* is the etiologic agent of Rocky Mountain Spotted Fever, which found in *D variabilis* (the dog tick) in Southeastern and Western states, and in *D andersoni* (the wood tick) in Rocky Mountain states.[16] Testing for both conditions involves enzyme-linked immunosorbent assay or polymerase chain reaction testing, and treatment is typically with oral or intravenous tetracycline.[16]

NEOPLASTIC NECK MASSES
Benign Neck Neoplasms

Pilomatrixoma
Hair follicle matrix cells may form pilomatrixomas, most typically in the suboccipital region or the posterior triangle[17] (**Fig. 19**). These lesions present as superficial, rock-hard, mobile neck masses and may have a bluish hue. They are slow growing, with a female preponderance.[1] Pilomatrixoma should be differentiated from epidermal and dermoid cysts; the latter two are less dense, deeper, and have normal overlying skin.[17] Pilomatrixomas slide freely over the underlying tissues; often, a "tent sign" can be elicited by stretching the skin over the tumor to feel the irregular surface of the mass.[17] Diagnosis can be made clinically and surgical excision is curative.

Lipomas
Lipomas are benign lesions and are rare in children. They consist of adipose tissue, and are painless, soft, and mobile on examination. These lesions can be excised surgically for functional or cosmetic purposes, if desired, because they may enlarge gradually.

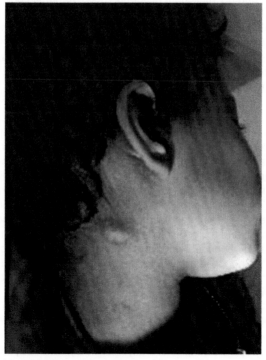

Fig. 19. A 5-year-old child with a pilomatrixoma.

Neural tumors

Benign neural tumors commonly involve cranial nerves and can present as isolated lesions or as part of a comprehensive syndrome. Neurofibromas (schwannomas), for example, may occur in autosomal dominant disorders.[1] Neurofibromatosis type 1 or von Recklinghausen disease is characterized by extensive nerve sheath tumor development and café-au-lait spots.[1] Children with neurofibromas of the head and neck should undergo imaging and genetic testing to rule out neurofibromatosis.[1]

MALIGNANT NECK NEOPLASMS AND METASTATIC LYMPHADENOPATHY

Malignant neck masses in children are uncommon. Several of the leading causes of metastatic cervical nodes in children are discussed below. Imaging modalities for the evaluation of acute lymphoblastic leukemia potentially malignant neck neoplasms involve ultrasound examination or contrast CT scanning with or without MRI. Treatment of pediatric malignant neck lesions typically consists of surgical excision and chemoradiation.[1]

Nasopharyngeal Carcinoma

Nasopharyngeal carcinoma is one of the most common nasopharyngeal tumors in young children.[18] It is distinguished from the adult form of the disease by its association with Epstein–Barr virus infection, undifferentiated histology, and high incidence of advanced locoregional compromise.[18] Painless, posterior cervical, metastatic nodes are typically seen with nasopharyngeal carcinoma.[18] It rarely occurs in children under 14 years of age.[18] Although enormous differences exist among races and geographic groups, nasopharyngeal carcinoma makes up 1% to 5% of all pediatric cancers and 20% to 50% of all primary malignant nasopharyngeal tumors in children.[18] There is a higher incidence in teenage males, those of Asian descent, and among children of Western industrial nations.[18] Patients may present with epistaxis and nasal obstructive symptomatology warranting evaluation with nasal endoscopy.[18] In children and adolescents, neoadjuvant chemotherapy and subsequent radiotherapy are preferred, but the best results are obtained with interferon-β, which is expensive and is not widely available in low-income countries.[18]

Lymphoma

Lymphoma is the most common malignant pediatric neck mass, reported to have a male predominance.[1] Non-Hodgkin lymphoma presents more commonly in children less than 10 years of age. Hodgkin lymphoma is more common in older children.[1]

Hodgkin lymphoma is a neoplastic disease of the lymphatic cell line and is distinguished histologically from non-Hodgkin lymphoma by its characteristic Reed-Sternberg cells.[19] Swollen, rubbery, nontender lymph nodes are frequently the most noticeable initial sign.[19] Histologic examination reveals Hodgkin and multinucleated Reed-Sternberg cells and multicolor lymphocytic reactions.[19] Anamnesis and clinical examination provide diagnostic indicators; staging is performed as in non-Hodgkin lymphoma with imaging, bone marrow aspiration, and histologic evidence of biopsied tissue.[19] Chemotherapy and, if applicable, radiotherapy are used as treatment options, according to the stage of the disease.[19]

Non-Hodgkin lymphomas are a heterogeneous group of neoplastic disorders of the lymphatic cell, which affects B-cell and T-cell lymphocytes.[19] The etiology is considered to be hereditary or acquired genetic defects leading to a mismatch of proliferation and apoptosis of cells in the lymphatic system.[19] Lymph node swelling and general symptoms such as fever, weight loss, and night sweats are the predominant manifestations.[19] Patients additionally often exhibit fatigue, weakness, and changes in blood count.[19] The swollen lymph nodes are usually firm and non-tender, and may be unilateral or bilateral.[19] Biopsy for histologic evaluation with special immune staining and bone marrow aspiration are necessary for diagnosis. Imaging is useful in staging the disease, including chest radiographs, CT scans, and ultrasound imaging of the neck, thorax, and abdomen.[19] Treatment is based on the stage and entity and may include chemotherapy, radiation, and/or antibody therapy.[19]

Neuroblastoma

Neuroblastoma is the most common head and neck malignancy in children less than 5 years of age, and it is the most common malignancy diagnosed during the first month after birth.[1] It can be associated with Horner syndrome and cranial neuropathies, as well as airway obstruction or dysphagia, because neuroblastomas arise in the neural crest progenitor cells of the sympathetic nervous system.[1] Treatment involves surgery and radiation for stage A disease (confinement to the nasal cavity). Stages B, C, or D disease (paranasal sinus involvement, extension to skull base, and distant metastasis including cervical lymph nodes, respectively) warrants surgery, radiation, and possibly postoperative chemotherapy.[1]

Rhabdomyosarcoma

Rhabdomyosarcoma is a highly malignant tumor of mesenchymal origin.[18] This neoplasm is the most common pediatric soft tissue sarcoma of the head and neck, and the second most common head and neck cancer. Rhabdomyosarcoma is typically encountered in children less than 10 years of age.[1] Upon biopsy, characteristic histologic indicators are eosinophilic cells and multinucleate giant cells.[18] In most cases, chemotherapy and radiation are initiated, and some cases additionally require surgical excision.[1]

Thyroid Malignancy

Thyroid nodules are infrequent in children. When present, they are more common in older children, and there is a high likelihood of malignancy.[1] Adenoma, papillary carcinoma (frequently associated with prior radiation therapy), follicular carcinoma, and medullary thyroid carcinoma can be distinguished via histopathological evaluation.[1] Multiple endocrine neoplasia syndrome type 2 is an autosomal-dominant, inherited condition that involves medullary thyroid carcinoma, pheochromocytoma, parathyroid hyperplasia (multiple endocrine neoplasia syndrome type 2A) and the addition of mucosal neuromas and marfanoid habitus (in multiple endocrine neoplasia syndrome type 2B).[1] Prophylactic thyroidectomy is the treatment of choice for multiple endocrine neoplasia syndrome type 2, as well as for patients with a history of head and neck radiation.[1]

Posttransplant Lymphoproliferative Disorder

After solid organ transplant, patients on immunosuppression may develop pathologic proliferations of lymphoid tissue, called posttransplant lymphoproliferative disorder.[1] This condition commonly presents with cervical lymphadenopathy and tonsillar hypertrophy, and is more common in children than adults.[1] Posttransplant lymphoproliferative disorder can range from lymphoid hyperplasia, such as tonsillar hypertrophy, to malignancy. Biopsy or tonsillectomy is confirmatory, and decreasing immunosuppressive medications is often indicated.[1]

OTHER

Additional etiologic considerations are worth mentioning. Castleman's disease is a proliferation of lymphatic cells commonly associated with HIV and human herpesvirus 8,1 and Rosai-Dorfman disease (sinus histiocytosis) is characterized by nonneoplastic proliferation of histiocytes in the sinusoids of lymph nodes and extranodal tissues.[20] Hematomas, which are localized collections of extravascular blood, may present after trauma or in association with underlying systemic disease. Uncommon infectious considerations include Lemierre syndrome, a septic thrombophlebitis of the internal jugular vein after infection of pharynx, which is associated with fusobacterium.[1] Lymphadenopathy may result from tularemia, which can be contracted via rabbits or rodents, although ticks can rarely be a vector.

Additional embryologic remnants of the head and neck to consider include auricular hillocks, which consist of ectopic cartilage deposits, found anywhere from the preauricular space, down the lateral neck, and even into the chest. Auricular hillocks are benign and do not require imaging, but are amenable to surgical intervention if they become infected or bothersome. Cervical bronchogenic cysts (foregut duplication cysts) result from anomalous foregut development, and are usually located in the thyroid or paratracheal region, or rarely in the suprasternal or supraclavicular location.[21]

Malignant salivary gland tumors in children primarily present in the parotid gland, with mucoepidermoid carcinoma being the most common.[1] These infrequently encountered entities are important to consider, but fall of outside of the scope of this article.

SUMMARY

Most pediatric neck masses encountered in primary care are benign, reactive lymph nodes that originate from common pediatric viral processes. In a pediatric otolaryngology practice, more unusual pathologies are encountered, such as embryologic anomalies, vascular lesions, or neoplasms. Normal lymph nodes are more easily palpable in children with thin necks, and benign-appearing lymph nodes in children are typically not considered for biopsy unless they are 3 cm or greater in size. Lesions that are larger or that have concerning features will ultimately need imaging and excisional biopsy for histopathologic confirmation of the diagnosis. A sound clinician understanding of anatomic neck spaces and common etiologies of pediatric neck masses can greatly reduce nonessential testing, cost, delay in treatment, and parental angst.

ACKNOWLEDGMENTS

The author would like to extend immense gratitude to Dr Stephen Early as her supervising physician and the sole pediatric otolaryngologist at The University of Virginia Medical Center. Thank you for hiring me twice, once in Florida, and then again 15 years later to join your practice at UVA in the Otolaryngology Head and Neck Surgery department. It has been a tremendous honor and privilege to have had the opportunity to work alongside you, truly one of the greatest minds and hearts of all time.

REFERENCES

1. Parikh S. Pediatric otolaryngology head and neck surgery clinical reference guide. San Diego (CA): Plural Publishing; 2014. p. 422–613.
2. Harish K. Neck dissections: radical to conservative. World J Surg Oncol 2005;3:21.

3. Meuwley J, Lepori D, Theumann N, et al. Multimodality imaging evaluation of the pediatric neck: techniques and spectrum of findings. Radiographics 2005;25(4): 931–48.
4. Mittal MK, Malik A, Sureka B, et al. Cystic masses of neck: a pictorial review. Indian J Radiol Imaging 2012;22(4):334–43.
5. Cahill AM, Nijs ELF. Pediatric vascular malformations: pathophysiology, diagnosis, and the role of interventional radiology. Cardiovasc Intervent Radiol 2011;34:691.
6. Craniofacial Development. Duke medicine embryology learning resources web site. Available at: https://web.duke.edu/anatomy/embryology/craniofacial/craniofacial. html Copyright © 2004-2011 Duke University School of Medicine. Accessed February 23, 2017.
7. Farhadi R, Sahebpour AA, Ghasemi M. Congenital midline cervical cleft: can it be treated in newborn? Iran J Pediatr 2012;22(4):547–50.
8. Adams A, Mankad K, Offiah C, et al. Branchial cleft anomalies: a pictorial review of embryological development and spectrum of imaging findings. Insights Imaging 2016;7(1):69–76. Available at: https://www.ncbi.nlm.nih.gov/pmc/articles/PMC4729717/. Accessed January 11, 2018.
9. Kaufman MR, Smith S, Rothschild MA, et al. Thymopharyngeal duct cyst: an unusual variant of cervical thymic anomalies. Arch Otolaryngol Head Neck Surg 2001;127(11):1357–60.
10. Shenoy V, Kamath MP, Hedge M, et al. Cervical thymic cyst: a rare differential diagnosis in lateral neck swelling. Case Rep Otolaryngol 2013;2013:350502.
11. Jishana J, Poduval JD. External laryngocele: points to remember. J Laryngol Voice 2013;3(2):67–9.
12. About hemangiomas and vascular birthmarks. EVMS Center for Hemangiomas and Vascular Birthmarks Web site. 2017. Available at: http://www.evms.edu/education/centers_institutes_departments/otolaryngology_ent/divisions/hemangiomas_and_vascular_birthmarks/. Accessed March 26, 2017.
13. Interdisciplinary Workgroup for Hemangiomas and Vascular Malformations web site. Available at: http://www.meduniwien.ac.at/haemangiom/index.php?page=1&lang=en Medical University of Vienna. Accessed May 26, 2017.
14. Orlow SJ, Isakoff MS, Blei F. Increased risk of symptomatic hemangiomas of the airway in association with cutaneous hemangiomas in a "beard" distribution. J Pediatr 1997;131:643–6.
15. Poirier VC, Ablin DS, Frank EH. Diffuse neonatal hemangiomatosis: a case report. AJNR Am J Neuroradiol 1990;11:1097–9. November/December 1990 0195-6108/90/1 106-1097 © American Society of Neuroradiology.
16. Bryant KA, Marshall GS. Clinical manifestations of tick-borne infections in children. Clin Diagn Lab Immunol 2000;7(4):523–7.
17. Danielson-Cohen A, Lin SS, Hughes A, et al. Head and neck pilomatrixoma in children. Arch Otolaryngol Head Neck Surg 2001;127(12):1481–3.
18. González-Motta A, González G, Bermudéz Y, et al. Pediatric nasopharyngeal cancer: case report and review of the literature. Cureus 2016;8(2):e497.
19. Lang S, Kansy B. Cervical lymph node diseases in children. GMS Curr Top Otorhinolaryngol Head Neck Surg 2014;13:Doc08.
20. Lima F, Barcelos P, Constancio A, et al. Rosai-Dorfman disease with spontaneous resolution: case report of a child. Rev Bras Hematol Hemoter 2011;33(4):312–4.
21. Kieran SM, Robson CD, Nose V, et al. Foregut duplication cysts in the head and neck presentation, diagnosis, and management. Arch Otolaryngol Head Neck Surg 2010;136(8):778–82.

Evaluation and Management of Adult Neck Masses

Trina M. Sheedy, MMS, PA-C

KEYWORDS

- Adult neck mass • Cervical lymphadenopathy • Primary care
- Oropharynx squamous cell carcinoma

KEY POINTS

- The incidence of malignancy is higher in adults older than 40 years old presenting with a neck mass.
- The cause of neck masses in the adult population in order of prevalence are as follows: neoplastic, infectious, and then congenital.
- Discerning pertinent questions to elicit a complete history, and comprehending the head and neck anatomy, in order to perform a meticulous examination, will be crucial skills for the primary care provider.
- Human papillomavirus–related oropharynx cancer is a well-recognized epidemic in Otolaryngology.

A new, persistent neck mass in an adult patient should be considered malignant until proven otherwise. Primary care providers and urgent care providers should keep malignancy at the top of their differential for an adult patient older than the age of 40 presenting with a neck mass, especially if that patient has particular risk factors. A thorough history and physical examination combined with a fundamental knowledge of head and neck anatomy can arm the primary care provider with all tools necessary to work up and properly diagnose a neck mass. Not all neck masses are neoplasms, but front-line providers should be familiar with the presentation and risk factors of those that are. The prognosis for those with malignancies is directly related to the stage, so early diagnosis is crucial.

ANATOMY

Before considering a differential diagnosis for a neck mass, the provider must be familiar with the anatomy of the head and neck. Anatomic landmarks are important to know, so that normal structures or viscera are not mistaken for abnormality. The

Disclosure Statement: None.
Head and Neck Surgical Oncology, Department of Otolaryngology–Head and Neck Surgery, University of California San Francisco, 1825 4th Street, 4th Floor, San Francisco, CA 94158, USA
E-mail address: Trina.Sheedy@ucsf.edu

Physician Assist Clin 3 (2018) 271–284
https://doi.org/10.1016/j.cpha.2017.11.006
2405-7991/18/© 2017 Elsevier Inc. All rights reserved.

physicianassistant.theclinics.com

tail of the parotid gland sits posterior and inferior to the angle of the mandible. The submandibular glands sit medial to the body of the mandible and extend inferiorly into the upper neck. The hyoid bone is only rarely palpable in the lateral aspects of a thin neck. The thyroid gland sits roughly two fingerbreadths below the thyroid cartilage (Adam's apple). In the posterior neck, the transverse processes of the spine may be palpable. Cervical lymphadenopathy is the presence of abnormal, usually enlarged, lymph nodes in the neck that can represent the immune response of a transient pathologic process or worse: the progression of a malignant disease.

Cervical lymph nodes comprise one-third of the body's lymphatic system and the drainage of the head and neck follows a predictable pattern. **Fig. 1** illustrates the direction of lymphatic flow from the vertex scalp down through the neck. The final lymph drainage from the head and neck collects into the right and left subclavian veins. In the left neck, the thoracic duct, bringing lymphatic fluid from the thorax and abdomen, also joins the left subclavian vein. Primary care literature typically groups the cervical lymph nodes into triangles. The author challenges the reader to consider an otolaryngology approach, which categorizes the neck into *levels* that more accurately reflect the nodal basins relevant to the head and neck subsites. The latest proposed anatomic classification, and the system most widely used among head and neck surgeons, is the Robbins Classification, which delineates the neck into 6 levels based on lymphatic drainage.[1] **Table 1** describes the significance of each level in the neck. A basic understanding of neck levels will aid in localizing the primary site of malignant or infectious disease in the presence of cervical lymphadenopathy.

It will benefit providers to be cognizant of the head and neck anatomic levels and the relationship between relevant systems including: the skin, sinonasal cavity, upper aerodigestive tract, endocrine system, neurovascular structures, and the lymphatic system. The lymphatic system drains the skin and all mucosal surfaces from the scalp

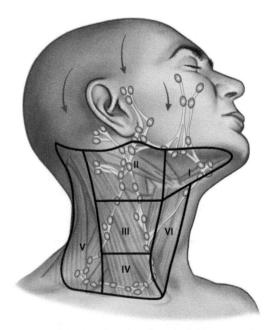

Fig. 1. Lymphatic drainage of the head and neck with delineation of Levels I-VI.

Table 1
Classification of neck levels and cervical lymph nodes

Robbins Classification	Clinical Location & Borders	Lymphatic Drainage Origination	Relevant Landmarks
Level I	IA, submental nodes	Midline: Mandible symphysis (S) to hyoid bone (I) and right anterior belly of digastric muscle to the left anterior belly (lateral borders)	Lower lip Anterior floor of mouth Tip of tongue	Submandibular glands
	IB, submandibular nodes	Body of mandible (S) to hyoid bone (I) and anterior belly of digastric muscle (M) to posterior border of submandibular gland (L)	Oral cavity[b] Anterior nasal cavity Skin of midface Submandibular gland	
Level II[a]	Upper jugular group	Mastoid process (S) to level of hyoid bone (I) and posterior border of submandibular gland (M) to posterior border of SCM (L)	Oropharynx[c] Hypopharynx Larynx Oral cavity	Tail of parotid gland Spinal accessory nerve Internal and external carotid artery and jugular vein Carotid bifurcation (transition of level II/III)
Level III[a]	Middle jugular group	Level of hyoid bone (S) to level of cricoid cartilage (I) and anterior border of SCM (M) to posterior border of SCM (L)	Oral cavity Nasopharynx Oropharynx Hypopharynx Larynx	Carotid bifurcation (transition of level II/III) Common carotid artery and jugular vein
Level IV[a]	Lower jugular group	Level of cricoid cartilage (S) to clavicle (I) and anterior border of SCM (M) to posterior border of SCM (L)	Hypopharynx Larynx Thyroid Cervical esophagus	Common carotid artery and jugular vein Virchow node
Level V	Posterior triangle group	Skull base where SCM and trapezius meet (S) to clavicle (I) and posterior border of SCM (M) to anterior border of trapezius (L)	Nasopharynx Oropharynx Skin of posterior scalp and neck	Spinal accessory nerve
Level VI	Anterior Compartment Group	Midline: Hyoid bone (S) to suprasternal notch (I) and right common carotid to left common carotid (lateral borders)	Thyroid Larynx Cervical esophagus	Thyroid gland Recurrent laryngeal nerves Parathyroid glands

Abbreviations: I, inferior; L, lateral; M, medial; S, superior; SCM, sternocleidomastoid muscle.
[a] II, III, IV jugulodigastric nodes are deep to the sternocleidomastoid muscle.
[b] Oral cavity includes: oral tongue, floor of mouth, mandibular gingiva, buccal mucosa.
[c] Oropharynx includes: soft palate, palatine tonsils, base of tongue.

and skull base to the larynx. Skin has a rich lymphatic supply so any abnormality of the scalp may result in lymphadenopathy in the parotid glands (intraparotid nodes) and level V. The paranasal sinuses play a major part in the healthy function of the respiratory system and can be affected by viral and bacterial pathogens. Resultant sinus inflammation may cause reactive lymphadenopathy in the lateral neck in level II. The upper aerodigestive tract includes the nasal cavity, nasopharynx, oral cavity, oropharynx, hypopharynx, and larynx; moreover, it is where the functions of eating, speaking, and breathing intersect. This upper aerodigestive region is lined with squamous mucosa and houses a collection of lymphoid tissue, which serves as the first line of defense against airborne and ingested pathogens. Depending on the subsite affected, related lymphadenopathy can manifest in levels I through V. Odontogenic infections should also be considered given that what was primarily a dental infection may expand into the neck or cause lymphadenopathy in level I. Reactive lymphadenopathy should correlate with a transient infection of the aerodigestive tract; however, if there are no signs or symptoms of infectious process, then the same region must be evaluated for a primary malignancy that has metastasized to regional lymph nodes. Other important viscera associated with the upper aerodigestive tract are the major and minor salivary glands that are responsible for exocrine functions in the oral phase of the digestive system. The salivary glands can be affected by infectious and inflammatory processes, but may also be a site of primary neoplasms. The endocrine glands of the neck, thyroid and parathyroids, lie in the low central neck and are common sites of benign and malignant lesions. Level VI is the most common first site of a nodal metastasis for thyroid cancer. Intimately related to the viscera and lymphatics of the neck, and also subject to pathology, are crucial neurovascular structures including carotid arteries, jugular veins, and cranial nerves.

PATIENT PRESENTATION

The age of a patient is the first factor a provider should consider when diagnosing a neck mass. Young adults, age 20 to 40, are more likely to present with a benign neck mass versus adults older than 40 years who are more likely to present with malignancy.[2] Besides the patient's age, a thorough history will be imperative. A provider must elicit the following details from the patient with a neck mass: onset, duration, characteristics, modifying factors, and associated symptoms of the mass. Additional history of exposures, travel, occupational hazards, substance abuse, and past medical/social/family history is pertinent. **Box 1** lists pertinent questions to consider when eliciting a history.

EXAMINATION

The presenting neck mass should be carefully examined by inspection and palpation. The location of the mass by neck level is most helpful for diagnosis, but at a minimum, a descriptor of midline versus lateral neck and upper versus lower neck should be noted. For example, localized disease of the major salivary glands would present in the unilateral or bilateral upper neck only. Infectious, inflammatory, and metastatic lymphadenopathy can all occupy the lateral neck: infectious or inflammatory is more likely to be bilateral, whereas early metastatic disease may be unilateral. Central neck masses could be congenital or neoplastic. Keeping in mind the soft tissue layers of the neck will help as well. A mass that is superficial within the dermis is likely an epidermal inclusion cyst (sebaceous cyst) or a cutaneous abscess. A soft mass in the subcutaneous tissue that moves with the skin could be a lipoma. A mass that is deep to the platysmal layer and mobile is likely an enlarged lymph node. A mass in

---

Box 1
Pertinent history questions

Onset: acute (days to weeks), subacute (weeks to months), or chronic (months to years)

Duration: constant or intermittent, fluctuating, growth pattern

Characteristics: pain, pressure, tenderness, skin changes

Modifying factors: worse or better with eating/swallowing, speaking/singing, change in position

Associated symptoms: globus, dysphagia, hoarseness, cough, hemoptysis, fever, chills, night sweats, weight loss

Exposures: cats, ticks, undercooked meat, recent travel, occupational hazards

Past medical history: skin cancer, previous neck surgery, autoimmune diseases, radiation therapy, immunocompromised

Social history: tobacco use, intravenous drug use, high-risk sexual behavior

Family history: thyroid disease/cancer, hyperparathyroidism, paraganglioma

---

the anterior low neck that moves with swallowing is likely a thyroid nodule. Delineating the location of a mass within the neck and its position relative to neighboring structures and organs should be assessed at the outset of the physical examination.

Further characteristics of the mass will narrow one's differential. Consider changes to the skin color, texture, and turgor. On palpation of the mass, note if it is ballotable, soft, rubbery, or firm. Is it tender to palpation? Is it freely mobile, limited in one direction, or fixed? Determine if there is only a single mass or if multiple masses are appreciated. If multiple masses, are they bilateral or unilateral? Although the patient's chief complaint may be a mass in the neck, the physical examination should incorporate inspection and palpation of the skin (scalp and face), ears, nose, oral cavity, oropharynx, major salivary glands, and thyroid gland. Any raised, ulcerative, or hyperpigmented lesions of the skin or nasal/oral mucosa could warrant biopsy. Oral cavity examination requires inspection of teeth, gingiva, and tongue. If not surgically absent, the palatine tonsils will be visible in the oropharynx. If they are erythematous or asymmetric in size, palpation of the palatine tonsils can be performed to rule out a firm mass. The salivary glands and thyroid gland should be symmetric and without nodules. The provider should make note of the patient's voice quality: whether it is rough, hoarse, or "hot-potato" sounding. A cranial nerve examination is important as well. Any abnormal finding could be related to the presenting neck mass.

DIAGNOSTIC WORKUP

Choice of diagnostic modalities is guided by a through history-taking and physical examination. Reasonable next steps may involve diagnostic ultrasound, computed tomography (CT) with contrast, or MRI; there may be reason to acquire a noncontrast CT or head/neck angiography as well. Imaging should be ordered based on a combination of clinical suspicion and what is available in the care setting to which the patient presents. Ultrasonography, which is not invasive nor does it involve radiation exposure, can be immensely telling. Neck ultrasound can differentiate solid versus cystic masses and confirm if a mass is within a gland (thyroid or salivary) or extraparenchymal. If a mass is palpable within the thyroid gland, confirmatory ultrasound may be the only imaging required. If it is clear from physical examination that a palpable mass is not within the viscera of the neck, but rather the soft tissue, then cross-sectional imaging will be the preferred and superior modality. If there is a strong clinical suspicion of malignancy based on *history*, like an older patient with B symptoms such as fever, night sweats, and weight loss who presents with a neck mass, or based on *examination*, like a patient with a palatine tonsil mass and ipsilateral neck lymphadenopathy, then a CT neck scan with contrast is recommended to rule out lymphoma and to rule out metastatic carcinoma respectively in these two examples. CT will provide anatomic detail of bone and the soft tissue of the neck and upper aerodigestive tract. Because of the magnetization, an MRI can provide much more soft tissue detail, resolution, and differentiation. If on first presentation the patient presents with cranial neuropathies, for example, an MRI will be critical to determine the cause of nerve injury.

Tissue biopsy is the gold standard for diagnosis of any neck mass. With the advent of fine needle aspiration (FNA), a diagnosis can usually be made on a cytologic sampling with almost no morbidity to the patient. Typically, neck mass diagnosis can be made based on interpretation of FNA without proceeding to excisional lymph node biopsy. Moreover, this is the preferred method for adults because of the higher rate of malignancy in this population. An incisional or excisional biopsy may confound tumor staging and result in more treatment. FNA done in combination with imaging guidance for needle placement into most the abnormal-appearing tissue will only enhance the diagnostic accuracy. Ultrasound-guided fine needle aspiration (USGFNA) of a neck mass, in the expert hand, can yield almost all diagnoses, whether that be reactive lymph nodes, benign neoplasms, metastatic lymphadenopathy, primary malignancy, infectious cause, inflammatory, or congenital mass.

CATEGORIZATION AND PREVALENCE

There are many ways to approach the categorization of adult neck masses: by prevalence, cause, acuity of onset, location in the neck, and presenting characteristics. Understanding this topic by its prevalence seems most relevant to clinical practice; however, the actual epidemiology of neck masses in adults is largely a mystery. The presentation of a palpable neck mass is a well-recognized chief complaint, but the incidence in the primary care and emergency care setting is unknown.[3] There is a paucity of retrospective studies that aim to define the epidemiology of neck masses in adults. One commonly cited study is a retrospective analysis of 82 patients, between 1982 and 1984, who underwent workup for unexplained lymphadenopathy. This paper concluded that the incidence of an adult presenting to a family practice provider with malignant cause of cervical lymphadenopathy was 1.1%. In addition, the investigators determined that adults older than the age of 40 have a 4% increased likelihood of malignancy.[4] In 1985, Williamson[5] published his retrospective analysis of 249 patients presenting to primary care for cervical lymphadenopathy; his findings were that only 3 patients (1.2%) were diagnosed with malignancy. However, only 36% of the 249 patients received a diagnosis at all. By contrast, nearly 30 years later, a Turkish study published in 2013 reviewed 630 patients (mean age 36.1 ± 6.80 years) with unexplained cervical lymphadenopathy *excluding* those with a known upper aerodigestive tract primary and known thyroid masses. Results showed that 23.3% were malignant neoplasms, 24.6% were benign neoplasms, 18.9% were congenital masses, and 33.5% were inflammatory masses.[6] Approximately one-quarter of these patients studied had malignancies *in addition* to those excluded from the study who already had known head and neck cancer. A 2015 study from the United Kingdom determined that primary care diagnoses of "lymphadenopathy" and "head and neck mass" had the greatest positive predictive values (18.6% and 4.6%, respectively) of leading to a diagnosis of lymphoma in patients ≥60 years old.[7] In addition, the 2015 edition of a staple ENT textbook, *Cummings Otolaryngology*, quotes that even with the exclusion of thyroid masses, there is an 80% chance of an adult neck mass being malignant.[2] It is likely time for a renewed epidemiologic study on the incidence of malignant neck masses in adults because the sources discussed above give a range of 1% to 80%.

Because the prevalence is not well understood, most literature approaches the topic by way of cause and classifies masses as neoplastic, infectious, or congenital. It is clear that in adults older than 40 years old the risk of malignancy is greater. Although cigarette smoking in the United States has fallen to the lowest rate in generations, the rising incidence of head and neck squamous cell carcinoma (SCC) caused by human papillomavirus (HPV) is an important factor. Providers evaluating adult neck masses should first consider malignancy because it is the most profound concern for a patient and has the greatest potential for morbidity. Following malignancy, the next important cause to rule out is an infectious cause. Last, congenital neck masses are far less common in adults, but they can present long after the childhood years. The following discussion is not a comprehensive list of neck mass causes, but a sampling of the ones most likely to be encountered.

NEOPLASTIC NECK MASSES

Neoplasms in the neck can arise from the structures and soft tissues within the neck; these lesions can be benign or malignant. More often, a malignant neoplasm in the neck is regional metastatic lymphadenopathy or, less commonly, a distant metastasis from a primary source below the diaphragm.[8] Using knowledge of nodal drainage patterns, the location of a neck metastasis can suggest the site of the primary tumor. Neoplasms can also arise within the thyroid or salivary glands. Lymphoma is a primary malignancy of the lymphatic system that is commonly identified by enlarged cervical nodes.

MALIGNANT NEOPLASMS

The 1988 estimate of 1.1% incidence of malignant cervical lymphadenopathy is likely outdated because of the discovery and rising incidence of HPV-related oropharynx cancer. Regardless of the overall incidence, 30% of adults who are diagnosed with head and neck cancer had cervical lymphadenopathy at their first clinic visit.[9] This statistic should sway providers to be vigilant about enlarged cervical lymph nodes in the adult population. In addition, a cystic neck mass requires careful diagnostic workup because nodal metastases of both HPV-related oropharynx cancer and thyroid cancer can present with cystic variants, which may be all too easily dismissed as a congenital lesion.

Metastatic Squamous Cell Carcinoma

The most common malignant neoplasm to present as a neck mass in an adult is metastatic squamous cell carcinoma with the primary site in the upper aerodigestive tract. In all patients older than the age of 40, SCC should be considered, and for those patients older than 60, the utmost suspicion should be of SCC.[9] Historically, head and neck SCC was related to heavy tobacco and alcohol use. However, it is now known that human papillomavirus has a propensity for causing SCC in the oropharynx; namely, arising within the palatine tonsils or the lingual tonsils embedded in the base of tongue. Moreover, HPV-caused oropharynx SCC occurs in adults who have nearly zero history of tobacco use. HPV is transmitted by oral sex to the oropharynx; current thought is that approximately 90% of oropharynx HPV infections are cleared from the body within 1 to 2 years, whereas roughly 10% persist. Persistent infections of HPV type 16 or 18 are a risk factor for oropharynx cancer development. Less than 1% of all persistent HPV oropharyngeal infections transform into malignancy, but with the ubiquity of HPV infections (both genital and oral) in sexually active young adults the incidence of HPV-related oropharynx cancer is rising. In the 1980s, only 16% of oropharyngeal tumors were HPV positive; in 2000, 73% were HPV positive.[10]

The patient with modern day head and neck cancer is typically a white man around the age of 55 to 65 with no past medical history and no tobacco history. HPV-related oropharyngeal cancers commonly present with a painless neck mass, which represents advanced metastatic disease. Associated symptoms may include throat pain, dysphagia, or globus sensation, but it is not uncommon for the patient to be completely asymptomatic. A typical male patient presents to primary or urgent care with a mass that "just appeared," which he noticed while shaving. Be wary of the reported acuity in this history; if the patient does not have other acute symptoms to suggest an infectious cause then the neck lesion is probably a malignancy. Another common presentation is a man with a several-month history of mild or progressive throat pain, for which he sees a primary care provider multiple times, but has no resolution of symptoms with antibiotic therapy. Again, the history does not correlate with infection because of the persistence of symptoms over several months. Physical examination should include careful palpation of the neck. Cervical metastatic lymphadenopathy from an oropharyngeal primary will present as a single or multiple firm, likely mobile, enlarged lymph nodes in level II or III. Diagnosis can be made on ultrasound-guided FNA. Otolaryngology management will include further workup with examination, endoscopy, and imaging to identify the primary site and staging.

Other Metastatic Cervical Lymphadenopathy

Cervical lymphadenopathy may represent metastatic disease from another primary cancer of the head and neck, such as thyroid cancer, cutaneous SCC, or melanoma. The history will have a subacute time course. Metastatic nodes from thyroid cancer will likely arise in the neck ipsilateral to the primary thyroid lesion. Location of a primary skin cancer will determine the location of neck metastases. The vertex scalp is a common location for both cutaneous SCC and melanoma and the predictable nodal pattern would suggest metastases in level V. Cutaneous SCCs of the anterior scalp or ears can also metastasize to lymph nodes within the ipsilateral parotid gland. A thorough skin cancer history should be taken along with careful inspection of the skin of the scalp, ears, and face. If there is no obvious skin primary, inspection for any pigmented lesion of mucosal nasal cavity and oral cavity should be considered for the rare mucosal melanoma. An enlarged single node in left level IV, Virchow node, should alert the provider to consider primary malignancies from breast, lung, or urogenital sources.

Lymphoma

Malignant neoplasms can also arise directly from the lymphatics or viscera of the neck. Lymphoma commonly presents with cervical lymphadenopathy and should be high on the differential of older adults or patients with constitutional symptoms, such as fever, weight loss, night sweats, or pruritus. Lymphoma is the second most common head and neck malignancy in the adult population. When presenting in the neck, lymphoma will likely be subacute in onset and can be located in the central or lateral neck. Confirmation of this diagnosis will involve FNA with flow cytometry.

Lymphoma is the one neck mass that may require an excisional biopsy for subtyping before treatment by a hematologist oncologist.

Thyroid Cancer

Thyroid nodules are commonly encountered in clinical practice with approximately 6% of people in iodine-rich countries having palpable thyroid nodules and another 20% to 60% of the population having nonpalpable thyroid nodules incidentally found on imaging.[11] A diagnostic ultrasound is the imaging test of choice for a palpable nodule or one found incidentally on cross-sectional imaging. Suspicious nodules should be biopsied. The American Thyroid Association reports that 7% to 15% of thyroid nodules are diagnosed as thyroid cancer.[11] The incidence of thyroid cancer almost doubled from 2009 to 2014, partly based on the improved detection of nodules and increased ease of diagnosis by FNA. Referral to an otolaryngologist is appropriate for management of benign and malignant thyroid nodules.

Salivary Gland Cancer

Salivary gland neoplasms can arise within any of the 3 major salivary glands, the parotid, submandibular, and sublingual glands, or in the minor salivary glands. Retrospective studies have shown that tumors arise most frequently in the parotid gland (73%), but only 14.7% of these are malignant. Conversely, the rate of tumor development in the submandibular glands is low and in the sublingual glands is rare; however, rates of malignancy in these glands are 37% and 85.7%, respectively.[12] Malignant salivary masses present as a single, unilateral, firm mass with limited mobility because of their location within the parenchyma of the gland. There is a long list of low-grade and high-grade malignant salivary gland neoplasms. Mucoepidermoid carcinoma followed by adenoid cystic carcinoma are the 2 most common. CT or MRI is warranted, along with ultrasound-guided needle biopsy. Cytologic results may not be definitive and oncologic resection by an otolaryngologist is needed for confirmatory diagnosis.

BENIGN NEOPLASMS

The neck can harbor neoplastic lesions that are benign yet not entirely innocuous. Benign neoplastic lesions have an indolent time course and will increase in size to varying degrees over many years. They may cause mass effect on critical structures of the neck, become cosmetically bothersome, or rarely cause systemic effects.

Thyroid Nodules and Thyroid Goiter

As mentioned previously, approximately 6% of the general population has palpable thyroid nodules, but by far most are benign follicular adenomas or benign thyroid cysts. Neck ultrasound and USGFNA can confirm benign abnormality. No intervention is warranted unless there is a change, such as nodule growth, or onset of compression symptoms, such as dysphagia, dyspnea, or voice changes. Benign nodules can be observed and ultrasound provides a facile modality for routine surveillance.

Four percent of the general population has thyroid goiters. A multinodular goiter (or nontoxic goiter) is a result of hypothyroidism, which effects women more than men and is more prevalent in older age. Autoimmune thyroiditis (Hashimoto) is the most common autoimmune disease, and the number one cause of a goiter. The patient's history will likely include a chronic timeline of a low central neck mass that in retrospect has been present for many years. Goiters are typically obvious: visible from across the room. To palpation, the thyroid gland will be diffusely enlarged, firm, and possibly tender. Goiters warrant surgical intervention based on presence of malignancy or compressive symptoms.

Salivary Gland Masses

By far the most common benign neoplasm of salivary glands is a pleomorphic adenoma (also called benign mixed tumor) arising from the parotid gland. These tumors are benign, but will grow over time and have the potential for malignant transformation. Because the facial nerve runs between the superficial and deep lobes of the parotid, surgical resection is preferred while the mass is relatively small in order to minimize risk of injury to the facial nerve. MRI is the preferred imaging study. FNA in the hands of an expert pathologist can correctly diagnose this tumor; however, complete surgical resection is recommended to confirm diagnosis.

Another commonly encountered benign salivary neoplasm is a Warthin tumor, which is associated with cigarette smoking. Warthin tumor can be confirmed on FNA and does not necessarily need to be surgically removed. Patients can develop several Warthin tumors. Surgical excision is reserved until the patient is symptomatic to minimize the possibility of repeat surgeries, which would increase the risk of complications, while not reducing the chance of developing yet another tumor.

Paraganglioma

Paragangliomas are a collection of benign neuroendocrine tumors that arise from the paraganglionic cells along parasympathetic nerves in the neck and skull base. The two most relevant, due to their location in the neck, are (1) carotid paragangliomas, which arise from the carotid blub, and (2) vagal paragangliomas, which arise from paraganglionic tissue associated with the vagus nerve. Patients may present with an asymptomatic mass or with complaints of pulsatile tinnitus, aural fullness, dizziness, or cranial neuropathies. Only 1% to 3% of paragangliomas are functional, causing paroxysmal hypertension, headache, flushing, and palpitations because of release of catecholamines.[8] On examination, these tumors will have limited cranial-caudal mobility in the direction of the nerve, but be freely mobile laterally. Because they are vascular tumors, MR angiography is the imaging study of choice. Catecholamine testing with 24-hour urine collection or plasma sample can rule out functional tumors.

Lipoma

Lipomas can arise anywhere on the body and their characteristics are the same in the neck as elsewhere, although the neck location may be more cosmetically bothersome. They are benign tumors arising from adipose tissue within the subcutaneous layer of the skin. Hence, on examination, they will move with the skin (versus roll around separately from the skin as will a lymph node). If desired by the patient, a lipoma on the head or neck could be excised by an otolaryngologist.

INFECTIOUS/INFLAMMATORY NECK MASSES

Most infectious or inflammatory causes of neck masses will be acute in onset and have other concurrent identifiable signs and symptoms. Viral illnesses certainly frequently impact the head and neck as do some bacterial processes. Influenza and streptococcal infections are common, whereas cat-scratch disease and tuberculosis are rare. The head and neck can be a site of localized inflammatory disease or involved in a more systematic process.

Viral Lymphadenopathy

Infectious causes that result in reactive cervical lymphadenopathy include numerous casually contracted viral upper respiratory illnesses (URIs), such as rhinovirus, adenovirus, and influenza. With common things being common, adults experience a self-limiting URI 2 to 4 times per year.[13] URIs can be associated with tender, enlarged, mobile, reactive bilateral cervical lymphadenopathy. It is expected that the acute symptoms of the URI will resolve in 1 to 2 weeks, but dissipation of the reactive nodes may take up to 6 weeks. If a node persists beyond this clinically reasonable timeframe, FNA might be warranted.

Other viral illnesses, beyond those localized to the upper respiratory system, may cause cervical lymphadenopathy in addition to generalized adenopathy. Such viruses include Epstein-Barr virus (EBV) and human immunodeficiency virus (HIV), both of which require intimate contact for transmission. There are numerous potential disease manifestations of EBV, including lymphoproliferative disorders and malignancy, but its most common primary presentation is mononucleosis. A patient with mononucleosis will typically experience acute onset of malaise, headache, fever, and tonsillopharyngitis along with enlarged, tender level II and III nodes. Treatment of mononucleosis is supportive and cervical lymphadenopathy is self-limiting. The evaluation and management of HIV and the multiple secondary infections that occur in immunocompromised persons are beyond the scope of this article.

Bacterial Lymphadenitis

Bacterial infections such as *Staphylococcus aureus* and Group A *Streptococcus* (GAS) are common causes of cellulitis, folliculitis, skin abscesses, and suppurative lymphadenopathy of the head and neck. GAS is a common bacterial cause of tonsillitis and painful level II and III lymphadenopathy. If a patient presents with infectious symptoms and signs of cellulitis or abscess of the head and neck skin, cervical lymphadenopathy would not be surprising. Management could include any combination of bacterial culture, incision and drainage, and antibiotic therapy.

Granulomatous Diseases

Other less common bacterial infections that may produce granulomatous reactions are cat-scratch disease and tuberculosis. These diseases are caused by *Bartonella henselae* and *Mycobacterium tuberculosis*, respectively. Cat-scratch disease is caused by infection with *B henselae* via transmission by a kitten or flea; lymphadenopathy will manifest near the site of inoculation. A history of contact with cats is positive in 90% of those diagnosed with cat-scratch disease.[14] Tuberculosis is transmitted by respiratory droplets and is primarily a pulmonary disease, but extrapulmonary infection is possible. Scrofula is the term for cervical lymphadenitis caused by *M tuberculosis*; this is very rare and most likely to be seen in an immunocompromised patient with HIV infection. These patients would require serologic workup and further evaluation by infectious disease specialists.

Although noninfectious, sarcoidosis is recognized as a systemic granulomatous disease. In sarcoidosis, granulomas form in affected organs and cause fibrosis of the tissue. The cause for this disease is unknown, but the most common persons affected are African American women. When sarcoidosis manifests in cervical lymph nodes, it can easily be identified on FNA. Management should include pulmonology workup and otolaryngology surveillance as needed.

Inflammatory

A truly acute, noninfectious process that is localized to the head and neck is sialadenitis. Inflammation of the gland and obstruction of saliva flow can be caused by a stone (sialolith) or stenosis of the duct. Symptoms of acute sialadenitis include episodic pain and swelling localized to site of affected gland when an individual begins to eat or salivate. The symptoms dissipate as quickly as a few minutes after eating, but may reoccur with every meal. Hydration and sialogogues are encouraged to mitigate painful symptoms. Secondary infections can occur requiring oral antibiotic therapy, or for severe infections, intravenous antibiotics. For some patients this is a one-time occurrence, but for others sialadenitis becomes a chronic problem for which patients may seek surgical intervention. To rule out a sialolith, a noncontrast neck CT is reasonable. Sialendoscopy, performed by specially trained head and neck surgeons, is a minimally invasive technique of cannulating the affected duct in order to remove the culprit of salivary duct obstruction.

Rarely, patients may have an autoimmune disorder such as Sjogren syndrome, which causes diffuse salivary gland inflammation and subsequent sialadenitis. Diagnostic imaging will reveal inflamed, heterogeneous bilateral parotid and submandibular glands. Individuals with Sjogren syndrome also complain of dry mouth and dry eyes. Management involves rheumatologic workup and treatment of underlying systemic disease.

CONGENITAL NECK MASSES

The least likely cause for an adult neck mass is congenital. "Low-flow" vascular malformations may present in adulthood. Thyroglossal duct cysts and branchial cleft cysts result from the incomplete obliteration of embryonic structures during fetal development. Included here, but not actually a congenital remnant, is a ranula.

Vascular Malformations

Most vascular anomalies are recognized in childhood, particularly hemangiomas and arteriovenous fistulas, which are "high-flow" vascular lesions that can have significant consequences. However, some adults present with "low-flow" vascular anomalies, including venous malformations and lymphatic malformations. Analysis of 18,073 individuals with contrast MRIs of the head revealed that the prevalence of venous anomalies increases with age.[15] If in the upper aerodigestive tract, patients may have complaints related to cosmesis or interference with breathing or swallowing. Vascular anomalies usually present as a soft, painless, lobulated, and possibly hyperpigmented (if venous) mass within the soft tissue of the neck or oral cavity. Surgical excision is not recommended, but rather sclerotherapy (to scar down and shrink the lesion) is the treatment of choice.

Thyroglossal Duct Cysts

Thyroglossal duct cysts are frequently identified as the most common congenital mass in the neck. They occur in the midline anterior neck arising from a persistence of the thyroglossal duct that does not involute during embryonic development. A URI usually precedes discovery of a thyroglossal duct cyst because it can become infected, enlarged, and thus noticeable, when before the URI, the patient was asymptomatic. Most patients desire removal of the mass for cosmetic reasons and most providers recommend surgery to avoid reinfection. An otolaryngologist will perform a Sistrunk procedure to remove the cyst and its track to prevent reformation.

Branchial Cleft Cysts

During embryonic development, there are pairs of branchial arches, and corresponding clefts, that develop as the precursor to head and neck structures. Failure of certain sinus tracts to obliterate give rise to malformations of the fetal head and neck, namely, branchial cleft cysts. Ninety-five percent of these anomalies present as a unilateral painless cystic mass in level II inferior to the angle of the mandible and along the anterior border of the sternocleidomastoid muscle.[2] Presentation has a bimodal age distribution with 75% identified in young adults aged 20 to 40.[16] Infections of these cysts can be treated with oral antibiotics before definitive treatment. Incision and drainage is contraindicated because the entire cyst and sinus tract need to be surgically excised to prevent recurrence.

Ranula

A mucocele is a benign collection of mucin (saliva) that can appear anywhere in the oral cavity arising from minor salivary glands within the mucosa. A ranula is a mucocele of the sublingual gland. A patient will present with a cystic submucosal mass in the left or right anterior floor of the mouth. A plunging ranula is a pseudocyst that contains extravasated mucin extending inferiorly from the sublingual gland into the soft tissue of the neck. Presentation will be a soft, painless mass in level I. To prevent recurrence, this requires surgical removal along with the sublingual gland.

SUMMARY

In conclusion, malignancy must not be missed; therefore, the evaluation of a neck mass in an adult should be a cautious one. The most probable diagnosis of a neck mass in adults (age over 40) is very different than in children and even young adults (ages 20–40). Providers should hone their history-taking and examination skills in order to distinguish between the various causes of a neck mass. Communicating pertinent information regarding the patient's age, risk factors, presentation, and physical characteristics to colleagues in radiology and cytopathology will increase the likelihood of coming to the correct diagnosis. Skepticism about a benign pathologic result is encouraged. Lastly, front line providers should not hesitate to consult with or promptly defer management to otolaryngology colleagues because most patients will require surgical intervention and a rising number will need comprehensive cancer care.

REFERENCES

1. Gregoire V, Lee N, Hamoir M, et al. Radiation therapy and management of the cervical lymph nodes and malignant skull base tumors. In: Flint PW, Haughey BH, Lund VJ, et al, editors. Cummings otolaryngology-head and neck surgery. 6th edition. Philadelphia: Saunders Elsevier; 2015. p. 1816–36.
2. Gregoire V, Lee N, Hamoir M, et al. Differential diagnosis of neck masses. In: Flint PW, Haughey BH, Lund VJ, et al, editors. Cummings otolaryngology-head and neck surgery. 6th edition. Philadelphia: Saunders Elsevier; 2015. p. 1767–72.
3. Learned KO, Malloy KM, Langer JE, et al. Adults with palpable neck mass: evidence-based neuroimaging. In: Medina LS, Sanelli PC, Jarvik JG, et al, editors. Evidence-based neuroimaging diagnosis and treatment. New York: Springer Science+Business Media; 2013. p. 641–77.
4. Fijten GH, Blijham GH. Unexplained lymphadenopathy in family practice. An evaluation of the probability of malignant causes and the effectiveness of

physicians' workup. J Fam Pract 1988;27(4):373–6. Available at: https://www.ncbi.nlm.nih.gov/pubmed. Accessed April 28, 2017.

5. Williamson HA. Lymphadenopathy in a family practice: a descriptive study of 249 cases. J Fam Pract 1985;20(5):449–52. Available at: https://www.ncbi.nlm.nih.gov/pubmed/?term=Williamson+HA.+J+Fam+Pract.+1985%3B20(5)%3A449%E2%80%9352. Accessed May 19, 2017.

6. Balikci HH, Gurdal MM, Ozkul MH, et al. Neck masses: diagnostic analysis of 630 cases in Turkish population. Eur Arch Otorhinolaryngol 2013;270(11):2953–8.

7. Shepard EA, Neal RD, Rose PW, et al. Quantifying the risk of non-Hodgkin lymphoma in symptomatic primary care patients aged ≥40 years: a large case–control study using electronic records. Br J Gen Pract 2015;65(634):e281–8.

8. Gregoire V, Lee N, Hamoir M, et al. Neoplasms of the neck. In: Flint PW, Haughey BH, Lund VJ, et al, editors. Cummings otolaryngology-head and neck surgery. 6th edition. Philadelphia: Saunders Elsevier; 2015. p. 1787–804.

9. Layfield LJ. Fine-needle aspiration in the diagnosis of head and neck lesions: a review and discussion of problems in differential diagnosis. Diagn Cytopathol 2007;35:798–805.

10. Fakhry C, D'Souza G. Discussing the diagnosis of HPV-OSCC: common questions and answers. Oral Oncol 2013;49(9):863–71.

11. Haugen BR, Alexander EK, Bible KC, et al. 2015 American Thyroid Association Management Guidelines for adult patients with thyroid nodules and differentiated thyroid cancer. Thyroid 2016;26(1):1–133.

12. Sunwoo JB, Lewis JS Jr, Tomeh C, et al. Malignant neoplasms of the salivary glands. In: Flint PW, Haughey BH, Lund VJ, et al, editors. Cummings otolaryngology-head and neck surgery. 6th edition. Philadelphia: Saunders Elsevier; 2015. p. 1258–80.

13. Haynes J, Arnold KR, Aguirre-Oskins C, et al. Evaluation of neck masses in adults. Am Fam Physician 2015;91(10):698–706.

14. Lin DT, Deschler DG. Neck masses. In: Lalwani AK, editor. Current diagnosis & treatment in otolaryngology—head & neck surgery. 3rd edition. New York: McGraw-Hill; 2012. p. 415–25.

15. Brinjikji W, El-Rida El-Masri A, Wald J, et al. Prevalence of developmental venous anomalies increases with age. Stroke 2017;48:1997–9.

16. Katabi N, Lewis JS. Update from the 4th edition of the World Health Organization classification of head and neck tumours: what is new in the 2017 WHO blue book for tumors and tumor-like lesions of the neck and lymph nodes. Head Neck Pathol 2017;11(1):48–54.

Ear, Nose, and Throat Manifestations of Sarcoidosis

Jennifer Johnson, MPAS, PA-C

KEYWORDS

- Sarcoidosis • Head • Neck • Great imitator • Granuloma • Lymph node
- Cervical lymphadenopathy

KEY POINTS

- It is crucial for detection of ear, nose, and throat (ENT) manifestations that practitioners consider sarcoidosis when constructing a differential diagnosis and selecting testing modalities for ENT symptoms with unusual presentations or that are refractory to treatment.
- Extrapulmonary manifestations of sarcoidosis are not uncommon, although they rarely occur in isolation.
- Of head and neck manifestations, the most common subsite is cervical lymph nodes.
- Initial misdiagnosis is common, necessitating tissue biopsy and radiologic imaging modalities in order to arrive at a correct diagnosis.
- Systemic corticosteroids are the mainstay of treatment for most ENT manifestations of treatment.

INTRODUCTION

Sarcoidosis is a multisystem inflammatory disease that can be difficult to diagnose. Although pulmonary structures are most commonly involved, sarcoidosis often involves structures of the head and neck. Initial misdiagnosis is common, necessitating tissue biopsy and radiologic imaging modalities in order to arrive at a correct diagnosis. This article will describe the case of a 25-year-old woman who presented to the clinic with a 2-month history of progressive otolaryngologic manifestations. Sarcoidosis has a tendency to mimic conditions with similar otolaryngologic presentations; therefore, it is important that practitioners consider sarcoidosis when constructing a differential diagnosis and selecting testing modalities. Considering a diagnosis of sarcoidosis is especially vital if symptoms are refractory to treatment or if presentation and examination findings are not consistent with more common

Conflict of Interest: None.
Physician Assistant Program, Rocky Mountain University of Health Professions, 122 East 1700 South, Provo, UT 84606, USA
E-mail address: jjohnson@rmuohp.edu

Physician Assist Clin 3 (2018) 285–295
https://doi.org/10.1016/j.cpha.2017.11.003
2405-7991/18/© 2017 Elsevier Inc. All rights reserved.

otolaryngologic diseases. This article will explore the challenges of diagnosis and treatment of sarcoidosis through a case study.

CASE STUDY

A 25-year-old woman presents to an otolaryngology clinic for evaluation of her mouth and throat. She is accompanied by her mother, who provides the patient's medical history. The patient has de Grouchy syndrome and is nonverbal. The patient's mother reports that the patient has experienced pain in the mouth and throat intermittently for the past 8 weeks. The current episode has persisted for 4 weeks. Associated symptoms include fever of 100.4 °F, reported oral lesions, and lymphadenopathy of the neck with tenderness. Mother denies skin rashes, diarrhea, nausea, nasal congestion, otalgia, rhinorrhea, coughing, dyspnea, or wheezing. Within the past 2 months, the patient has been seen by her dentist, primary care provider, and 2 emergency department physicians. Per the patient's mother, radiographs of the neck, jaw, and dentition are normal. She was diagnosed with hand, foot, and mouth disease (HFMD) and has subsequently been treated with courses of amoxicillin clavulanate, valacyclovir, and prednisone. However, her symptoms did not respond to these treatments and she has continued to worsen. The patient's mother is adamant that something else is causing her daughter's symptoms and expresses frustration with the lack of answers.

On examination, the patient's head is normocephalic and atraumatic. Her tympanic membranes, external auditory canals, and external ears are within normal limits bilaterally. No rhinorrhea is noted, and no nasal mucosa edema is present. On examination of the oropharynx, no oral lesions are visible, and tonsils are within normal limits. Poor dentition is noted, and dental caries are present. Wharton and Stensen ducts are patent with normal salivary flow bilaterally, with no intraductal masses or stones palpable. Palpation of the neck reveals scattered anterior lymphadenopathy bilaterally, more prominent on the right side superiorly. The right submandibular gland is mildly enlarged on palpation. Cardiovascular and pulmonary findings are within normal limits on physical examination.

After discussing findings and options with the patient's mother, she elects to proceed with computed tomography (CT) of the neck with intravenous contrast. The scan reveals extensive bilateral enhancing jugular chain adenopathy with the largest lymph nodes visible at the angle of the right mandible (**Fig. 1**) and irregular enhancement of the right submandibular gland with a pattern suspicious for infiltration by the disease affecting the adjacent markedly enlarged lymph nodes (**Fig. 2**). The radiologist notes that the appearance of the lymphadenopathy is most consistent with lymphoma. Subsequently, the largest lymph node is removed via an excisional biopsy, and pathology confirms granulomatous lymphadenitis with morphologic features highly suggestive of sarcoidosis; malignancy is ruled out.

BACKGROUND

As illustrated by this case study, sarcoidosis has a long-recognized reputation as a difficult-to-diagnose disease and is often referred to as the great imitator, especially with regard to extrapulmonary manifestations. Sarcoidosis can occur in almost any organ system and usually involves more than 1 organ.[1] Sarcoidosis was initially described by Jonathan Hutchinson in 1869 as a dermatologic condition. Over time, sarcoidosis gained recognition as a multisystem disorder with a high incidence of pulmonary abnormalities.[2] In addition to the lungs and skin, other organs commonly affected by sarcoidosis include heart, kidneys, eyes, liver, central nervous system, peripheral nervous system, lymph nodes, and upper respiratory tract.

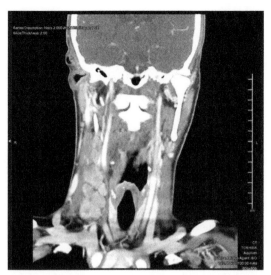

Fig. 1. Coronal image of enhanced neck CT. Extensive bilateral enhancing jugular chain aden-opathy with the largest lymph nodes seen at the angle of the right mandible in a 25-year-old female.

EPIDEMIOLOGY AND ETIOLOGY

Sarcoidosis may be found worldwide, although the highest prevalence has been re-ported in Scandinavian countries.[3] Higher prevalence also occurs in Ireland and in the southeast coastal region of the United States (**Fig. 3**).[4] Sarcoidosis is slightly more prevalent in women, and in the United States it is more prevalent in African

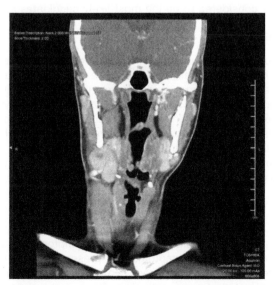

Fig. 2. Coronal image of enhanced neck CT. Irregular enhancement of the right submandib-ular gland with a pattern suspicious for infiltration by the disease affecting the adjacent markedly enlarged lymph nodes in a 25-year-old female.

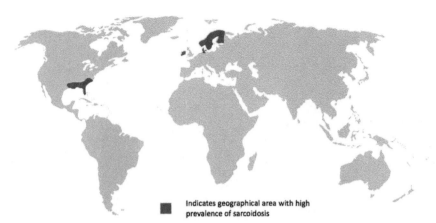

Indicates geographical area with high
prevalence of sarcoidosis

Fig. 3. Though sarcoidosis is found worldwide, higher prevalence is reported in Scandinavia, Ireland, and in the southeast coastal region of the United States.

Americans. Most cases of sarcoidosis are diagnosed in otherwise healthy individuals in the second and third decades of life, although a second peak occurs in women during the sixth decade. The prevalence in North America and Europe ranges from 10 to 80 cases per 100,000 population.[4]

The exact etiology of sarcoidosis is unknown, but likely multifactorial. The National Heart, Lung, and Blood Institute (NHLBI) assembled a multicenter ACCESS study to gain insight into this question.[5] However, a clearly defined etiology was not discovered. Given that disease clustering is observed both familially and geographically, it is likely that an environmental or microbial exposure triggers the disease in genetically susceptible individuals.[6] Recent studies have explored the possibility of a microbial trigger in sarcoidosis, with mycobacteria and *Propionibacterium acnes* considered to be the most likely candidates at this time.[7,8]

PATHOPHYSIOLOGY

Sarcoidosis is caused by a cell-mediated immune response. The distinctive features of sarcoidosis include CD4+ T cell infiltration at the site of inflammation and the formation of noncaseating granulomas. Antigens from unidentified environmental or microbial exposures interact with CD4+ T cells and activated monocytes accumulate. Cytokines are released, including interleukin (IL)-2, interferon γ, and tumor necrosis factor (TNF).[3] This immune response leads to creation of macrophage-giant cells, which mass together and wall-off the antigen, resulting granuloma formation.[9] This granuloma may resolve acutely or progress to a chronic disease state, with the latter occurring in 20% of patients.[3]

SIGNS AND SYMPTOMS

The presentation of sarcoidosis is variable and ranges from asymptomatic with incidental findings to nonspecific constitutional symptoms, to severe disease with organ failure. Pulmonary symptoms are present in 90% of patients and commonly include dry cough and dyspnea (**Box 1**).[4] Common nonspecific constitutional symptoms include fatigue, arthralgia, fever, and weight loss.[10] Because these common presenting symptoms are vague, correct diagnosis can easily require multiple clinic visits and often takes up to 12 months from the time of

---

Box 1
Common presenting symptoms of sarcoidosis are often nonspecific and vague

Dry cough

Dyspnea

Fatigue

Fever

Weight loss

Arthralgias

Adenopathy

Cutaneous lesions

Ocular symptoms

---

symptom onset.[3] The occurrence of ocular or cutaneous manifestations may lead to an increased clinical suspicion for sarcoidosis and more prompt diagnosis based on the presence of anterior uveitis or easily visible cutaneous lesions, respectively.[11]

DIAGNOSIS

Once clinical suspicion for sarcoidosis has been aroused, imaging of the involved organs is the initial step in the diagnostic process. The exception is cutaneous lesions, which are typically biopsied upon discovery. The most common initial imaging study is a chest radiograph to evaluate persistent pulmonary symptoms, and expected findings include bilateral hilar lymphadenopathy and pulmonary infiltration. Other common forms of imaging used to evaluate extrapulmonary manifestations of sarcoidosis include ultrasound, computed tomography (CT), MRI, and positron emission tomography (PET) scans. Selection of the most appropriate form of imaging should be based on location of patient symptoms and suspected organ involvement, which will be discussed on an organ system basis, as follows. It should be noted that ultrasound has been found to have poor specificity for sarcoidosis.[12]

The next step in the diagnostic process is biopsy of the most accessible abnormal tissue.[4] Pathology evaluation of a tissue sample obtained through biopsy is considered the gold standard for the diagnosis of sarcoidosis.[4,13] Tissue biopsy will accomplish 2 things: confirm the diagnosis of sarcoidosis and aid in ruling out other conditions, including granulomatous diseases, malignancies, and microbial causes such as tuberculosis. Additional tests for consideration to rule out other granulomatous diseases include:

- Complete blood cell (CBC) count with differential
- Comprehensive metabolic panel (CMP)
- PPD
- cANCA
- CD4+/CD8+ ratio
- Serum angiotensin-converting enzyme
- Pulmonary function tests
- Bronchoalveolar lavage
- Kveim-Siltzbach reaction

EAR, NOSE, AND THROAT MANIFESTATIONS

Extrapulmonary manifestations of sarcoidosis are not uncommon, although they rarely occur in isolation. It is estimated that 10% to 15% of patients with sarcoidosis demonstrate head and neck manifestations.[11] Of head and neck manifestations, the most common subsite is the cervical lymph nodes.[14] Other subsites discussed in this article include the larynx, sinonasal region, salivary gland, ear, and pituitary gland. Ocular manifestations will also be discussed, though they are not typically classified as ENT manifestations.

CERVICAL LYMPH NODES

Cervical lymphadenopathy resulting from sarcoidosis represents a diagnostic challenge to providers, particularly in the absence of pulmonary or other organ involvement. Although cervical lymphadenopathy is the most common head and neck manifestation of sarcoidosis, only 1.7% of all head and neck lymphadenopathy is caused by sarcoidosis.[15,16] Sarcoid lymphadenopathy presents as enlarged, tender lymph nodes (**Table 1**). Imaging tests, such as a CT scan of the neck with contrast, can increase clinical suspicion of sarcoidosis in the presence of hilar node enlargement and calcifications while simultaneously aiding in selection of the most accessible node for biopsy. Sarcoidosis can often be distinguished from other causes of lymphadenopathy during excisional biopsy and pathology evaluation by characteristic sharp demarcation, acid-fast staining, and a lack of central necrosis.[17,18]

Table 1
Locations and symptoms of ENT manifestations of sarcoidosis

Location	Symptoms
Cervical lymph node	Lymph node enlargement Tenderness
Larynx	Dysphonia Dysphagia Globus sensation Upper airway obstruction
Sinonasal region	Nasal congestion Rhinitis Nasal polyps Epistaxis Frequent nasal crust formation Anosmia
Salivary gland	Unilateral, painless enlargement of salivary gland Dryness of the mouth Facial nerve palsy
Ear	Sensorineural hearing loss Facial nerve paralysis Vestibular dysfunction
Eye	Anterior uveitis Intermediate uveitis Posterior uveitis
Pituitary gland	Diabetes insipidus Gonadotropic deficiency TSH deficiency Hyperprolactinemia

An interesting case study recently reported an instance of sarcoidosis isolated to a solitary cervical lymph node, with immunohistochemistry revealing abundant expression of tumor necrosis factor (TNF)-α in the granuloma.[19] Another case identified sarcoidosis in a cervical lymph node that was initially misdiagnosed as a parathyroid adenoma in a patient with unexplained hypercalcemia.[20] Hypercalcemia occurs in 2% to 63% patients with sarcoidosis as a result of uncontrolled synthesis of 1,25-Dihydroxyvitamin D3 by macrophages, which in turn leads to increased resorption of calcium in the bone and increased absorption of calcium in the intestine.[20–23] If high clinical suspicion for sarcoidosis in a cervical lymph node exists and the diagnosis is unsure, it may be prudent to consider evaluation of serum calcium levels and expression of TNF-α in the granuloma. Systemic corticosteroids are considered the mainstay of treatment for cervical lymphadenopathy resulting from sarcoidosis.

LARYNX

Sarcoidosis of the larynx has an estimated incidence of 0.33% to 2.1% and tends to occur in the supraglottic region, specifically at the site of the epiglottis.[24,25] Other common sites in the supraglottic region include aryepiglottic folds, false vocal folds, and arytenoid cartilages.[24] Presenting symptoms may include dysphonia, dysphagia, or globus sensation. A primary concern with sarcoidosis of the larynx is the potential for obstruction of the upper airway, which could become severe and potentially life-threatening. Flexible fiberoptic laryngoscopy (FFL) and CT scan with contrast are beneficial in the diagnosis of sarcoidosis of the larynx and allow for direct visualization and determination of the extent of the disease. FFL typically reveals a pale, swollen epiglottis with multiple nodules visible. Roughly 10% of laryngeal sarcoidosis patients will experience spontaneous remission.[26] Treatment modalities for laryngeal sarcoidosis include systemic corticosteroids, immunosuppressive agents, steroid injection, and CO_2-laser excision.[24,25]

SINONASAL

Sinonasal sarcoidosis is rare and likely underdiagnosed due to nonspecific presenting symptoms, occurring in roughly 1% of sarcoidosis patients.[27] The most frequent signs and symptoms include nasal congestion, rhinitis, nasal polyps, epistaxis, frequent nasal crust formation, and anosmia.[27] Common sites of occurrence include the nasal septum, inferior turbinates, paranasal sinuses, nasal bone, cartilage, and subcutaneous tissue.[28,29] A thorough head and neck examination should be performed, including nasopharyngoscopy. Mucosal nodules of the septum and turbinates are the most suggestive features found on maxillofacial CT, with biopsy required for definitive diagnosis.[30] Additional findings in more advanced disease include nasal bone and cartilage destruction, resulting in an accompanying saddle nose deformity. It should be noted that 1 study found PET/CT provides a better diagnostic sensitivity (100%) in addition to complete morphofunctional mapping of active inflammatory sites of sinonasal sarcoidosis.[30] First-line therapy for sinonasal sarcoidosis consists of endoscopic surgery with biopsy for histologic confirmation and systemic corticosteroids. Additional therapies include topical intranasal steroids, as well as biologic therapies such as methotrexate and azathioprine.[27]

SALIVARY

Salivary gland manifestations of sarcoidosis are rare, with parotid gland involvement occurring in roughly 2% of patients with sarcoid.[31] The most common presenting symptom of sarcoidosis of the salivary glands is unilateral, painless enlargement of a salivary gland. Bilateral enlargement of the salivary glands has been reported in the literature.[32] Salivary gland manifestations of sarcoidosis can occur in either the parotid glands or submandibular glands, and rarely in the sublingual salivary glands. Other presenting symptoms can include dryness of the mouth or even facial nerve palsy from parotid sarcoid involvement. There have been reports indicating that most cases of submandibular sarcoidosis occur in women.[33] Heerfordt syndrome is a form of salivary gland sarcoidosis associated with parotid gland enlargement, fever, lacrimal gland enlargement, uveitis, bilateral hilar adenopathy, and cranial nerve involvement, specifically the facial nerve.[4] It should be considered when evaluating a patient with suspected sarcoidosis of the parotid glands. As with other manifestations, contrast enhanced CT of the neck may further increase clinical suspicion for sarcoidosis of the salivary glands, and tissue biopsy should be obtained for histologic confirmation. Discussion of treatment options for salivary gland manifestations is limited in the literature; however, several case reports document favorable responses to systemic corticosteroids. It is not uncommon for unilateral salivary gland sarcoidosis to be misdiagnosed as a benign tumor on CT, such as a pleomorphic adenoma. As a result, sarcoidosis may not be discovered until after surgical removal of the salivary gland when operative pathology evaluation is pursued.

OTOLOGIC

Otologic manifestations of sarcoidosis are exceedingly uncommon and rarely discussed in the literature, and the exact incidence is unknown. Presenting symptoms may include sensorineural hearing loss, facial nerve paralysis, and vestibular dysfunction. Sudden-onset, fluctuating sensorineural hearing loss has been reported.[34] Otologic sarcoidosis can also involve the skin and cartilage of the external ear, the external auditory canal, middle ear structures, and the temporal bone. The temporal bone should be evaluated using high-resolution CT scan if involvement is suspected. A burst and taper of systemic corticosteroids is the initial treatment choice if rapid hearing loss is involved. Referral to a neurotologist for surgical exploration and management may be necessary if the middle ear structures or temporal bone demonstrate significant involvement.

OCULAR

Although not typically categorized as a head and neck manifestation, it is important to recognize ocular sarcoidosis, as it accompanies salivary gland enlargement and cranial nerve involvement in Heerfordt syndrome. Ocular manifestations of sarcoidosis are common. One study found that ocular manifestations were present in 21% of sarcoidosis patients at the time of initial presentation, and anterior uveitis was the most frequent ocular manifestation.[35] Intermediate and posterior uveitis also occur, but are less common. Clinical findings associated with anterior uveitis of ocular sarcoidosis origin include bilateral, chronic granulomatous iridocyclitis with keratic precipitates and iris nodules.[35] Biopsy of ocular structures is usually avoided whenever possible, as chest radiograph and CT are often positive for pulmonary manifestations, with less morbidity involved in lung biopsy. Ocular sarcoidosis warrants an ophthalmology consult, and an ophthalmologist should be integrated into the multidisciplinary treatment team. Treatment of chronic anterior uveitis includes topical corticosteroids, topical cycloplegics, regional corticosteroid injections and implants, systemic corticosteroids, systemic immunosuppressive agents, and biologic agents.[36]

PITUITARY GLAND

Although pituitary disorders are often outside of the scope of practice of most otolaryngologists, hypothalamo-pituitary (HP) manifestations of sarcoidosis warrant discussion, because they mimic several endocrine disorders and often initially present as such. This includes thyroid disorders, which are often encountered in otolaryngology practices. HP manifestations of sarcoidosis are rare, constituting less than 1% of sella turcica lesions, and usually involve the anterior pituitary gland.[37] One retrospective chart review identified the median age of diagnosis as 31.5 years.[37] Presenting symptoms of these patients are associated with endocrine disorders.[10] The most common presenting endocrine abnormalities are diabetes insipidus, gonadotropic deficiency, TSH deficiency, and hyperprolactinemia.[37] MRI is the imaging study of choice and may reveal pituitary stalk thickness or involvement of the infundibulum or pituitary gland itself.[37] Systemic corticosteroids, specifically prednisone, are the treatment of choice for the majority of patients with HP manifestations. Abnormalities found on MRI may improve or resolve with corticosteroid treatment; however, most endocrine defects are irreversible despite systemic corticosteroid treatment.[37]

SUMMARY

Sarcoidosis is a multisystem disorder that presents a diagnostic challenge for otolaryngology providers, as the initial presenting symptoms are nonspecific. ENT extrapulmonary manifestations are rare and therefore often overlooked. The 25-year-old woman presented in the aforementioned case study was subsequently referred to a rheumatologist for further evaluation, and a diagnosis of sarcoidosis was confirmed. The rheumatologist assumed management of the patient, and she was treated with oral corticosteroids. Otolaryngology follow-up was recommended on an as-needed basis, as indicated by subsequent testing or should additional ENT manifestations occur. At the time of this article, she is still being monitored by rheumatology. Because of the nature of most ENT manifestations of sarcoidosis, a multidisciplinary treatment approach may be necessary and is in the best interest of the patient. Systemic corticosteroids are the mainstay of treatment for most manifestations of sarcoidosis, but they are often used in conjunction with topical or intralesional steroids, surgical treatment, immunosuppressive agents, and other therapies. It is crucial that otolaryngology providers consider sarcoidosis when constructing a differential diagnosis and selecting testing modalities for ENT symptoms with unusual presentations or that are refractory to treatment.

REFERENCES

1. Tchernev G. Cutaneous sarcoidosis: the 'great imitator'. Am J Clin Dermatol 2006; 7(6):375–82.
2. Spagnolo P. Sarcoidosis: a critical review of history and milestones. Clin Rev Allergy Immunol 2015;49(1):1–5.
3. Baughman RP, Lower EE. Sarcoidosis. In: Kasper D, Fauci A, Hauser S, et al, editors. Harrison's principles of internal medicine. 19th edition. New York: McGraw-Hill; 2014.
4. Chen ES, Moller DR. Chapter 54. Sarcoidosis. In: Imboden JB, Hellmann DB, Stone JH, editors. Current diagnosis & treatment: rheumatology. 3rd edition. New York: McGraw-Hill; 2013.
5. Semenzato G. ACCESS: a case control etiologic study of sarcoidosis. Sarcoidosis Vasc Diffuse Lung Dis 2005;22(2):83–6.

6. Iannuzzi MC, Rybicki BA. Genetics of sarcoidosis: candidate genes and genome scans. Proc Am Thorac Soc 2007;4(1):108–16.
7. Eishi Y. Etiologic aspect of sarcoidosis as an allergic endogenous infection caused by propionibacterium acnes. Biomed Res Int 2013;2013:935289.
8. Grunewald J, Eklund A. Role of CD4+ T cells in sarcoidosis. Proc Am Thorac Soc 2007;4(5):461–4.
9. Schwartzbauer HR, Tami TA. Ear, nose, and throat manifestations of sarcoidosis. Otolaryngol Clin North Am 2003;36(4):673–84.
10. Badhey AK, Kadakia S, Carrau RL, et al. Sarcoidosis of the head and neck. Head Neck Pathol 2015;9(2):260–8.
11. Mrowka-Kata K, Kata D, Lange D, et al. Sarcoidosis and its otolaryngological implications. Eur Arch Otorhinolaryngol 2010;267(10):1507–14.
12. Teymoortash A, Werner JA. Parotid gland involvement in sarcoidosis: sonographic features. J Clin Ultrasound 2009;37(9):507–10.
13. Braun JJ, Kessler R, Constantinesco A, et al. 18F-FDG PET/CT in sarcoidosis management: review and report of 20 cases. Eur J Nucl Med Mol Imaging 2008;35(8):1537–43.
14. Chen H-C, Kang B-H, Lin Y-S, et al. Sarcoidal granuloma in cervical lymph nodes. J Chin Med Assoc 2005;68(7):339–42.
15. Dash GI, Kimmelman CP. Head and neck manifestations of sarcoidosis. Laryngoscope 1988;98:50–3.
16. Chumakov FI, Khmeleva RI. Head and neck lymph node lesions. Vestn Otorinolaringol 2002;6:27–9.
17. Asano S. Granulomatous lymphadenitis. J Clin Exp Hematop 2012;52(1):1–16.
18. Newman LS, Rose CS, Maier LA. Sarcoidosis. N Engl J Med 1997;336:1224–34.
19. Kwon YS, Jung HI, Kim HJ, et al. Isolated cervical lymph node sarcoidosis presenting in an asymptomatic neck mass: a case report. Tuberc Respir Dis (Seoul) 2013;75(3):116–9.
20. Calò PG, Pisano G, Tatti A, et al. Cervical lymph node sarcoidosis mimicking a parathyroid adenoma: a clinical case. Clin Med Insights Case Rep 2013;6: 159–63.
21. Krikorian A, Shah S, Wasman J. Parathyroid hormone-related protein: an unusual mechanism for hypercalcemia in sarcoidosis. Endocr Pract 2011;17(4):e84–6.
22. Sharma OP. Vitamin D, calcium, and sarcoidosis. Chest 1996;109(2):535–9.
23. Falk S, Kratzsch J, Paschke R, et al. Hypercalcemia as a result of sarcoidosis with normal serum concentrations of vitamin D. Med Sci Monit 2007;13(11):CS133–6.
24. Duchemann B, Lavolé A, Naccache JM, et al. Laryngeal sarcoidosis: a case-control study. Sarcoidosis Vasc Diffuse Lung Dis 2014;31:227–34.
25. Tsubouchi K, Hamada N, Ijichi K, et al. Spontaneous improvement of laryngeal sarcoidosis resistant to systemic corticosteroid administration. Respirol Case Rep 2015;3(3):112–4.
26. Bower JS, Belen JE, Weg JG, et al. Manifestations and treatment of laryngeal sarcoidosis. Am Rev Respir Dis 1980;122:325–32.
27. Kirsten A-M, Watz H, Kirsten D. Sarcoidosis with involvement of the paranasal sinuses - a retrospective analysis of 12 biopsy-proven cases. BMC Pulm Med 2013;13:59.
28. Joseph B, Vyloppilli S, Sayd S, et al. Sinonasal sarcoidosis of the maxillary sinus and infraorbital nerve: a case report. J Korean Assoc Oral Maxillofac Surg 2015; 41(4):217–21.
29. Braun JJ, Gentine A, Pauli G. Sinonasal sarcoidosis: review and report of fifteen cases. Laryngoscope 2004;114:1960–3.

30. Braun J-J, Imperiale A, Riehm S, et al. Imaging in sinonasal sarcoidosis: CT, MRI, 67Gallium scintigraphy and 18F-FDG PET/CT features. J Neuroradiol 2010;37(3): 172–81.

31. Ungprasert P, Crowson CS, Matteson EL. Clinical characteristics of parotid gland sarcoidosis: a population based study. JAMA Otolaryngol Head Neck Surg 2016; 142(5):503–4.

32. Sharma T, Joshi D, Khurana A, et al. Bilaterally enlarged parotids and sicca symptoms as a presentation of sarcoidosis: pivotal role of aspiration cytology in diagnosis. J Cytol 2015;32(4):281–3.

33. Shah UK, White JA, Gooey JE, et al. Otolaryngologic manifestations of sarcoidosis: presentation and diagnosis. Laryngoscope 1997;107(1):67–75.

34. Hybels RL, Rice DH. Neuro-otologic manifestations of sarcoidosis. Laryngoscope 1976;86(12):1873–8.

35. Bodaghi B, Touitou V, Fardeau C, et al. Ocular sarcoidosis. Presse Med 2012; 41(6 Pt 2):e349–54.

36. Pasadhika S, Rosenbaum JT. Ocular sarcoidosis. Clin Chest Med 2015;36(4): 669–83.

37. Langrand C, Bihan H, Raverot G, et al. Hypothalamo-pituitary sarcoidosis: a multicenter study of 24 patients. QJM 2012;105(10):981–95.

Primary Hyperparathyroidism

Jeffrey M. Robin, MSHS, PA-C

KEYWORDS

- Hyperparathyroidism • Hypercalcemia • Ectopic parathyroids • Parathyroidectomy
- Nephrolithiasis • Bone densitometry • Localization studies

KEY POINTS

- Primary hyperparathyroidism is one of the leading causes of outpatient hypercalcemia.
- Serum calcium is controlled by parathyroid hormone, which achieves homeostasis by acting on bone resorption, kidney absorption, and intestinal absorption of calcium.
- Primary hyperparathyroidism can affect bone integrity and kidney function.
- Parathyroidectomy is the only cure for primary hyperparathyroidism. Preoperative assessment attempts to identify how many parathyroid glands may be involved and their anatomic location.
- Criteria for surgical intervention is based primarily on the degree of bone and kidney involvement.

INTRODUCTION

Primary hyperparathyroidism (PHPT) is one of the leading causes of hypercalcemia in the outpatient setting. Most individuals with hypercalcemia caused by PHPT are asymptomatic and are diagnosed incidentally during routine laboratory work without the classic symptoms of "stones, groans, moans, and psychiatric overtones."[1] This article provides a comprehensive review of parathyroid embryology and anatomy, physiology, the updated guidelines for the work-up and management of PHPT, presurgical preparation, and surgical and medical treatment modalities. Other causes of hyperparathyroidism, including secondary or tertiary hyperparathyroidism, and hereditary or genetic syndromes, including multiple endocrine neoplasia conditions, are not covered in this article.

PARATHYROID EMBRYOLOGY AND ANATOMY

There are 4 parathyroid glands, so named based on their anatomic relationship to the thyroid gland (left superior and inferior, right superior and inferior); however, the exact locations can vary considerably.[2] Each gland weighs less than 50 mg and measures

Disclosures: None.
Head and Neck/Endocrine Surgery, Swedish Cancer Institute, 1221 Madison Street, 15th Floor, Seattle, WA 98104, USA
E-mail address: jeffrey.robin@swedish.org

Physician Assist Clin 3 (2018) 297–312
https://doi.org/10.1016/j.cpha.2017.11.001
2405-7991/18/© 2017 Elsevier Inc. All rights reserved.

physicianassistant.theclinics.com

about 3 to 8 mm in length.[3] Their color has been described as tan, brown, or caramel, in contrast with the fatty tissue that can also be found in these locations, which is usually more yellow. The left and right inferior thyroid arteries (ITAs) provide the blood supply to the parathyroid glands.

During the 5th to 12th week of embryologic development, the parathyroid glands form from the endoderm of the third and fourth pharyngeal pouches.[4] The superior parathyroid glands originate from the fourth pharyngeal pouch and the inferior parathyroid glands from the third pharyngeal pouch. The inferior glands travel with the thymus, with the migration of the 2 structures often diverging as the thymus enters the mediastinum. This longer distance of embryologic travel for the inferior glands is the cause of variability and asymmetry in their location anywhere along this tract: the angle of the mandible (rare), the carotid sheath, along the thyrothymic ligament, and into the mediastinum.

The superior parathyroid glands can be found in a more predictable location compared with the inferior parathyroids. The left and right superior parathyroid glands are symmetric in location 80% of the time and, in the inferior parathyroid glands, 70% of the time.[5] Akerström and colleagues[5] are credited with the observation that the superior glands tend to be in a 2-cm diameter area centered 1 cm above the intersection of the recurrent laryngeal nerve (RLN) and the ITA.[3] The superior glands are also commonly found dorsal and lateral to the RLN, whereas the inferior glands are found ventral and medial. Wang's[6] publication in 1976 reported that, despite this anatomic variability, 77% of superior glands are found at the cricothyroid joint and 43% of inferior glands are located anterior to or at the posterolateral surface of the lower pole of the thyroid. One-third of inferior parathyroids are found within the pathway of the thyrothymic ligament (**Fig. 1**A).

Despite the higher incidence of anatomic variability of normal inferior parathyroid glands, adenomas originating from superior parathyroid glands have a higher incidence of ectopic location compared with inferior parathyroid adenomas. Up to 40% of superior parathyroid adenomas are ectopic and can be found in paraesophageal or retroesophageal, prevertebral, or upper mediastinal locations[7] (**Fig. 1**B).

CALCIUM REGULATION AND PARATHYROID PHYSIOLOGY

Serum calcium is one of most tightly regulated ions in the body, and is largely managed by the parathyroid glands.[8] About 99% of the body's calcium is in bone. Roughly half of serum calcium is free or ionized, which is biologically active. Forty percent is bound to proteins, mainly albumin. The remaining 10% is complexed calcium: bound to various anions. Besides being the main element for bone and cartilage mineralization, calcium is also used at the intracellular level for muscle contraction, neurotransmitter release, the coagulation cascade, and endocrine and exocrine secretion.[9]

Parathyroid hormone (PTH) is an 84-length amino acid peptide synthesized in parathyroid gland chief cells. PTH secretion is regulated by serum ionized calcium concentration. On the parathyroid cell surface, there are calcium sensing receptors (CaSR), which, when activated by calcium, suppress PTH secretion via a negative feedback loop.

PTH acts to increase the plasma concentration of calcium in 3 ways: (1) it stimulates bone resorption, (2) it augments active renal calcium absorption within the kidney, and (3) it enhances intestinal calcium absorption by promoting the formation of 1,25-dihydroxyvitamin D_3 [1,25$(OH)_2D_3$][9] (**Fig. 2**).

Parathyroid Hormone Action on Bone

To state that PTH increases bone resorption and osteoclast activity resulting in increased serum calcium level would be telling only half of the story about the role of PTH in bone. PTH stimulates both bone resorption and bone formation.[2]

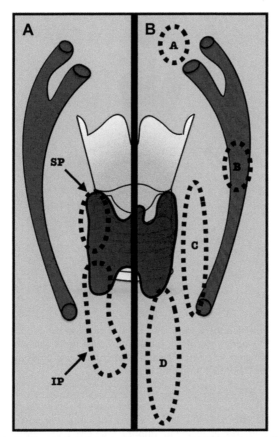

Fig. 1. (*A*) Normal distribution of the superior parathyroid (SP) and the inferior parathyroid (IP) glands. (*B*) Potential sites for ectopic parathyroid glands/adenomas; A, angle of mandible; B, carotid sheath, C, paraesophageal/prevertebral; D, mediastinal. (*Courtesy of J. Robin, PA-C and P. Robin.*)

PTH acts on osteoclast precursors, stimulates osteoclast maturation, and decreases osteoclast apoptosis. PTH receptor activation can also cause osteocytes to release calcium from bone, a mechanism called osteocytic osteolysis.[2] Osteoclasts do not have PTH receptors. Instead, PTH increases the synthesis of 2 surface proteins (M-CSF [macrophage colony-stimulating factor] and RANKL [receptor activator of nuclear factor kappa-B ligand]), which then bind to tumor necrosis factor receptors on both osteoclast precursors and mature osteoclasts.[2]

There are multiple in-vivo and in-vitro studies that have shown both direct and indirect actions of PTH on increased bone production. Similar to the action on osteoclasts, PTH increases osteoblast precursors, increases the number of active osteoblasts, and decreases the rate of osteoblast apoptosis.[10–13] Bone densitometric studies show that PTH is catabolic on cortical bone but anabolic on trabecular bone.[2] Bone mineral densitometry is further discussed later.

Parathyroid Hormone Action on the Kidney

PTH has renal influence in stimulating calcium reabsorption. The majority of filtered calcium is reabsorbed in the proximal convoluted tubule, with 20% in the loop of Henle

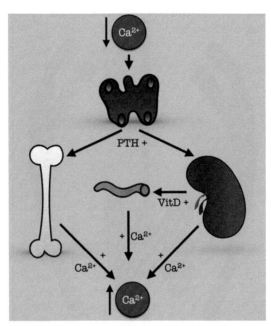

Fig. 2. PTH and calcium feedback loop. PTH acts to increase the plasma concentration of calcium by stimulating bone resorption, increasing active renal calcium absorption within the kidney, and enhancing intestinal calcium absorption by promoting the formation of 1,25-dihydroxyvitamin D_3 (VitD). (*Courtesy of* F. Robin.)

and 10% by the distal tubule.[9] With an increase in calcium reabsorption, it may be surmised that this would result in lower urinary calcium level. However, with PHPT, increased urinary calcium excretion occurs as a consequence of an increase in the filtered load of calcium from the serum.

Parathyroid Hormone, Vitamin D, and Action on the Intestine

The active form of vitamin D, $1,25(OH)_2D_3$, is synthesized by the proximal tubules of the kidney, which are activated by PTH. This form of vitamin D acts directly on the enterocytes of the small intestine to stimulate intestinal calcium absorption. Vitamin D enhances calcium absorption by 30% to 40%, whereas, without vitamin D, only 10% to 15% of dietary calcium is absorbed.[14] In hypovitaminosis D, intestinal calcium absorption is diminished and PTH levels increase in an attempt to maintain normal serum calcium levels and to increase $1,25(OH)_2D_3$ synthesis. This process may result in secondary hyperparathyroidism, which is beyond the scope of this article. However, individuals with synchronous PHPT and hypovitaminosis D show more pronounced effects of PHPT than those with PHPT alone.[15]

PRIMARY HYPERPARATHYROIDISM

PHPT occurs when 1 or more of the parathyroid glands become hypercellular and/or enlarged, resulting in excessive production of PTH. The regulating negative feedback loop that controls PTH and serum calcium level is impaired and any normal parathyroid tissue becomes suppressed, causing synchronous increased serum calcium and parathyroid levels. A single parathyroid adenoma is the cause in 80% to 85% of patients with PHPT. Four-gland hyperplasia causes 15%. Double adenomas cause 2% to 3% of PHPT, whereas parathyroid carcinoma causes less than 1%.[7] On the cellular level, a parathyroid adenoma cannot be distinguished from parathyroid hyperplasia because both present with similar cytologic features.[16]

In the United States, more than three-quarters of patients diagnosed with PHPT are asymptomatic and lack the classic symptoms of stones, bones, and groans, as first described by Fuller Albright in 1930.[1] The documented incidence of PHPT increased dramatically in the 1970s after the arrival of the automated serum autoanalyzer.[2] The peak incidence of PHPT occurs between the fifth and sixth decades of life; however, it may present at any age. It affects women more than men by roughly 3:1.[2]

As previously described, PTH acts on the receptors in the kidney and bone to increase levels of serum calcium. Over time, the kidneys become at risk for nephrolithiasis and bones can lose density, increasing the risk of fracture.

Diagnosis

When a concern for PHPT arises, either because of patient symptoms or from an incidental finding of random increased serum calcium level, the work-up begins with additional laboratory studies:

- Serum calcium/ionized calcium (serum calcium range is 8.6–10.2 mg/dL; ionized calcium range is 4.4–5.4 mg/dL [1.1–1.35 mmol/L])
- Second-generation (intact) or third-generation (whole) PTH assay (intact PTH range is 15–65 pg/mL)
- Serum creatinine (range, 0.57–1.00 mg/dL)
- Vitamin D (25(OH)D) (range, 30.0–100.0 ng/mL)

Differential Diagnosis of Hypercalcemia

The 2 most common causes for hypercalcemia in the outpatient setting are PHPT and malignancy. With PHPT, the PTH level is increased or in the upper limit of normal range. Hypercalcemia secondary to malignancy results in a suppressed PTH level.

Lithium and thiazide diuretic-induced hypercalcemia also presents with increased PTH levels. Withholding lithium and thiazide diuretics for 3 months should allow for serum calcium and PTH normalization. If increased calcium and PTH levels persist after medication discontinuation, then the patient has PHPT.[2]

Familial hypocalciuric hypercalcemia (FHH) is a benign autosomal dominant condition caused by a mutation in CaSR (discussed earlier) that also presents with increased serum calcium and PTH levels. It is a rare condition but it is important to differentiate FHH from PHPT because treatment is not indicated and failure to diagnose it may lead to inappropriate attempts at intervention.

Urine calcium tests can be helpful for determining whether a patient has FHH or PHPT. The 24-hour urine calcium level in FHH is classically low (<100 mg/d) and, although with PHPT it is high (>200 mg/d), hypercalciuria is not pathognomonic for either condition. A urine calcium/creatinine clearance ratio (UCCR) can also be measured. If the UCCR is 0.01 to 0.02 then gene mutation testing (CaSR and others) for FHH should be initiated. UCCR greater than 0.02 is likely to indicate PHPT.[17] **Fig. 3** provides an algorithm for the work-up of hypercalcemia.

Manifestations of Primary Hyperparathyroidism

In the early twentieth century, about 25% of patients with PHPT presented with advanced bone disease from osteitis fibrous cystica with brown tumors (**Fig. 4**) and

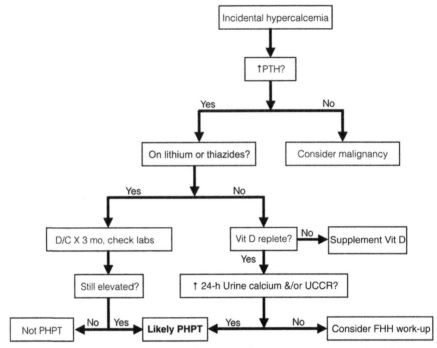

Fig. 3. Algorithm for hypercalcemia work-up. D/C, discontinue. (*Courtesy of* J. Robin, PA-C.)

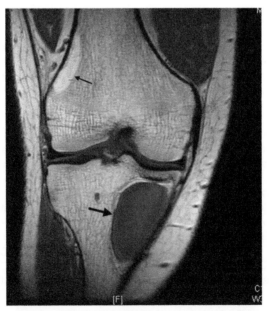

Fig. 4. Coronal MRI of brown tumor of the medial proximal right tibia (*dark arrow*). There are also additional changes of the distal femur caused by severe hyperparathyroidism (*thin arrow*). This patient presented with a PTH level of 560 pg/mL and serum calcium level of 12.4 mg/dL. His adenoma was 6.5 cm and 16 g.

almost 60% had nephrolithiasis.[18] Now, less than one-fifth of patients with PHPT have symptomatic kidney stones and only 2% have bone disease because of more facile diagnostic capabilities.[2]

Bone

Increased bone resorption in PHPT seems to occur at a greater magnitude in cortical bone as opposed to cancellous or trabecular bone. Bone mineral densitometry (BMD) via dual energy x-ray absorptiometry (DEXA or DXA) scans is the gold standard modality for evaluating bone disease in PHPT. Typically, demonstration of bone loss is greatest at the forearm (distal one-third of radius), a site that is almost totally composed of cortical bone, and least at the lumbar spine, a site with a large component of trabecular bone.[19] However, lumbar spine DEXA value may overestimate bone strength in PHPT, bringing the diagnostic accuracy of DEXA in lumbar spine assessment into question.[20] There are other modalities gaining attention in endocrinology that measure quantitative bone loss and can identify decreased trabecular/lumbar BMD that DEXA alone has been unable to detect.

Trabecular bone score (TBS) is an analysis that can be applied to, and is readily available from, DEXA images.[20] TBS can enhance the ability of DEXA to identify patients with and without fractures and to predict osteoporotic fractures and fracture risk. In PHPT, TBS may also identify trabecular abnormalities not captured by lumbar spine BMD. With these findings, TBS could become a helpful clinical tool for skeletal assessment in PHPT.[20]

Evaluating fracture risk in PHPT, particularly in mild cases, is fraught with conflicting evidence. Because PTH has an effect on both bone resorption and formation, bone densitometry alone may not reflect bone integrity as clearly as it can in postmenopausal women and in patients receiving osteoporosis assessment,[2] which suggests that other bone qualities beside density influence fracture risk. However, there are no studies that predict fracture risk in the context of PHPT based on DEXA or other quantitative modalities.[20]

Kidney

Nephrolithiasis has always been the commonly noted complication of PHPT; however, the incidence has greatly changed since the 1970s. Until the late 1960s, kidney stones were seen in 60% to 80% of cases of PHPT (**Fig. 5**). Now, because of improved

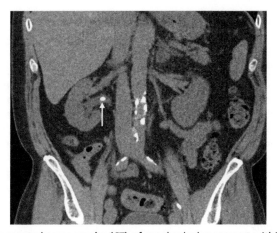

Fig. 5. Coronal computed tomography (CT) of renal calculus present within the right renal pelvis (*white arrow*) measuring 7.5 × 4.5 mm in a patient with PHPT with a PTH level of 83 pg/mL, serum calcium level of 10.3 mg/dL, and 24-hour urine calcium level of 444 mg/d. There are also incidental atherosclerotic calcifications of the abdominal aorta.

diagnostics and therapeutics, the frequency has decreased to about 15% to 20%.[21] PHPT accounts for about 3% of all cases of nephrolithiasis.[9]

Other renal manifestations of PHPT include hypercalciuria and nephrocalcinosis.[2] Hypercalciuria is seen in about 40% of patients with PHPT. Nephrocalcinosis is direct mineralization of renal tissue. Hypercalciuria is diagnosed on 24-hour urine calcium collection. Nephrocalcinosis is a radiologic diagnosis, the gold standard imaging modality being computed tomography (CT). Ultrasonography (US) and plain films can also be used.

Cardiovascular

Hypercalcemia has been associated with coronary artery disease, hypertension, and carotid plaques, but the role of hyperparathyroidism on these cardiovascular conditions remains unclear. Studies evaluating the possible cardiac manifestations of hyperparathyroidism have not been able to consistently show improvement in, or reversal of, these conditions after parathyroidectomy.[20]

Neurocognitive

Although fatigue, irritability, depression, and cognitive impairment are common findings seen with PHPT, studies showing postoperative improvement of these symptoms compared with controls are inconsistent.[20]

SURGICAL INDICATIONS

Parathyroidectomy is the only available treatment to cure PHPT. Once the diagnosis is made, symptomatic patients (history of fractures, osteoporosis, severe bone pain, nephrolithiasis) should be offered surgery. However, for the other 75% of patients with PHPT who are asymptomatic, an appropriate work-up to find evidence of renal or skeletal involvement should be undertaken.

The Fourth International Workshop on the Management of Asymptomatic Primary Hyperparathyroidism was held on September 19 to 21, 2013, in Florence, Italy. These updated guidelines, as revised from the prior (third) workshop in 2008, are reviewed here. Patients need to meet only 1 of the criteria presented later to be candidates for parathyroidectomy.

Increased Serum Calcium Level

Serum calcium levels greater than 1.0 mg/dL of the upper limit of normal (**Table 1**).

Bone Compromise

DEXA scans are recommended when evaluating asymptomatic patients for potential surgical intervention (see **Table 1**). Because cortical bone loss seems to be more severe than trabecular loss in PHPT, it is important to include the forearm during DEXA scans. A T score of less than −2.5 at any site (lumbar spine, total hip, femoral neck, or distal one-third radius) is an indication for surgery. Use of Z score is recommended in men less than 50 years old and in premenopausal women.[20]

DEXA scans should not be used for evaluation of vertebral fracture. Instead, to screen for vertebral fracture, which is an indication for surgery, vertebral imaging by radiograph, CT, or TBS is recommended.

Renal Manifestations

The International Workshop has updated the renal recommendations for treatment of asymptomatic PHPT from the previous recommendations in 2008 (see **Table 1**). Now, having a creatinine clearance less than 60 mL/min, a 24-hour urine calcium level

Table 1
Comparison of previous and new guidelines for surgery in asymptomatic primary hyperparathyroidism

	2008	2013
Measurement of Serum Calcium Level	>1.0 mg/dL upper limit of normal	>1.0 mg/dL upper limit of normal
Skeletal	BMD by DEXA: T score <−2.5 at any site[a]	A. BMD by DEXA: T score <−2.5 at lumbar spine, total hip, femoral neck, or distal one-third radius B. Vertebral fracture on imaging[a]
Renal	eGFR<60 mL/min	A. Cr clearance <60 mL/min B. 24-h urine Ca >400 mg/d and increased stone risk C. Presence of nephrolithiasis or nephrocalcinosis on imaging
Age (y)	<50	<50

Abbreviation: eGFR, estimated glomerular filtration rate.
[a] The use of Z score instead of T score is recommended when evaluating BMD in premenopausal women and men younger than 50 y.

greater than 400 mg/d, increased stone risk by biochemical stone analysis of the 24-hour urine evaluation, or presence of nephrolithiasis or nephrocalcinosis (by radiograph, US, or CT) are each indications for surgery.

Biochemical stone analysis determines whether the stone risk is caused by calcium-derived stones (vs uric acid, struvite, or cystine) and whether stone-inhibitory products are present (urine citric acid or urine magnesium).[22]

The risk of radiation with renal imaging, particularly with radiograph and CT, may be challenging to justify to a patient or insurance company, especially when the patient is asymptomatic. It is more cost-effective and less invasive to start with the 24-hour urine collection and thereafter decide whether imaging would be beneficial, pending results.

Cardiovascular Abnormalities

Assessment for cardiovascular abnormalities is not recommended during PHPT evaluation, nor should cardiovascular manifestations be considered in decisions regarding surgery.[20]

Neurocognitive Compromise

Some patients with neurocognitive dysfunction benefit from surgical intervention. However, it is not possible at this time to predict which patients with neuropsychological complaints or cognitive issues will improve after successful parathyroid surgery; therefore, neuropsychiatric and cognitive dysfunction should not be considered during decision making for surgery for PHPT.[20]

MEDICAL MANAGEMENT

Asymptomatic patients who do not meet the surgical criteria discussed earlier or those who are not considered surgical candidates can be followed medically. Annual serum calcium and creatinine testing is recommended. BMD should also be measured every 1 to 2 years.[23]

It might seem appropriate to limit patients' dietary intake of calcium in the context of PHPT. However, there is some evidence that, by restricting dietary calcium, PTH levels may continue to increase. Increasing dietary calcium of 500 to 1000 mg/d can suppress PTH in some patients with PHPT.[24]

Patients should also be replete in vitamin D. However, those with increased levels of 25(OH)D can develop increased hypercalciuria.[2]

Alendronate is the most studied bisphosphonate in treatment of PHPT. It can increase the BMD of the lumbar spine and hip, but does not change the serum calcium level.[2]

Cinacalcet is a calcimimetic compound that activates cloned CaSR and reduces serum calcium levels by inhibiting PTH secretion.[9] PTH levels also decrease but typically do not enter the normal range.

PHPT is first and foremost a surgical disease. Any attempt to treat this disease medically because of poor surgical candidacy or lack of surgical criteria should be undertaken by an endocrinologist.

SURGICAL INTERVENTION

Once the decision to pursue surgical intervention is made, referral to an experienced endocrine surgeon is strongly recommended. The surgeon should have experience with minimally invasive parathyroidectomy, 4-gland parathyroid exploration, and bilateral neck dissection.

Because most cases of PHPT are caused by a single adenoma (80%–90%), minimally invasive, single-gland excision has become a more common method of surgical treatment compared with the traditional 4-gland exploration or bilateral neck dissection. For both techniques, first-time parathyroid surgery yields a success rate of 95% to 98%.[25,26] Minimally invasive surgery has some features that can be appealing for patients; smaller incision, shorter operative time, possible same-day discharge, and shorter recovery time. Contraindications to minimally invasive surgery include suspicion for, or diagnosis of, multigland disease, prior neck surgery, or revision parathyroidectomy. Even if preoperative studies strongly suggest a single adenoma, surgeons should always be prepared to convert from a minimally invasive procedure into a 4-gland exploration if intraoperative findings reveal possible multigland disease. This conversion may include exploring the upper mediastinum, carotid sheath, or paraesophageal and prevertebral spaces (discussed earlier). The possibility for an extensive neck exploration is an important preoperative conversation to have with the patient.

If minimally invasive surgery is going to be pursued, then preoperative localization studies are performed. Imaging should not be used for the diagnosis of PHPT.

Localization Studies

Parathyroid imaging tests include nuclear imaging with sestamibi technetium-99m (Tc99m), US, and four-dimensional CT (4DCT). MRI is used less frequently.

Sestamibi

Sestamibi Tc99m is a lipophilic molecule that is taken up by cells with high concentrations of mitochondria. Parathyroid adenomas and hyperplastic parathyroid glands have an increased uptake compared with normal parathyroid glands.[27] Also, there is a prolonged washout of Tc99m from the parathyroid cells compared with the thyroid gland. This prolonged washout allows these scans to be performed in dual phase; images are captured at 20 to 30 minutes and at 2 hours after injection of the radiotracer.[28] The abnormal parathyroids show persistent uptake in the delayed images at 2 hours (**Fig. 6**). Sestamibi has a sensitivity of approximately 88% for localizing

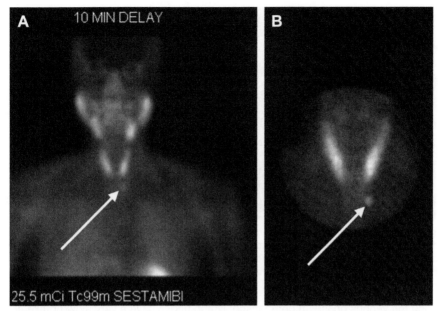

Fig. 6. Sestamibi Tc99m study revealing a left mediastinal parathyroid adenoma (*arrows*).

single adenomas.[29] False-negative results are typically caused by early washout of the radiotracer, multiple hyperplastic parathyroid glands, presence of thyroid nodules, or a multinodular goiter.[27]

Ultrasonography

US is an effective, low-cost, radiation-free imaging modality that can be performed not just by radiologists but also by parathyroid surgeons. Successful detection of a single parathyroid adenoma by US alone ranges in the literature from 51% to 96%.[30] There are multiple articles reporting the additional benefit of surgeon-performed US for parathyroid localization, ranging from 87% to 90%.[28,30–33] The American Association of Endocrine Surgeons Guidelines for Definitive Management of PHPT state that cervical US performed by an experienced parathyroid sonographer is the least costly imaging modality and, when combined with sestamibi or 4DCT, is the most cost-efficient strategy.

Parathyroid adenomas on US appear as hypoechoic (dark), ovoid structures often within the central neck. In-office, surgeon-performed US also provides real-time, three-dimensional visualization of the surrounding anatomy (thyroid, carotids, internal jugular veins, esophagus), which allows preoperative planning (**Fig. 7**).[27] Failure to identify parathyroid adenomas, or disadvantages of US, include operator dependence, patient obesity, presence of goiter or multiple thyroid nodules, multigland disease, and presence of ectopic disease.

Four-dimensional computed tomography

In 4DCT, the images are captured based on the timing of contrast administration. Parathyroid glands, and hyperplastic parathyroid tissue in particular, have a rapid wash in (arterial phase) and washout (venous phase) of contrast material compared with the thyroid gland and lymph nodes. There are 3 phases of imaging: noncontrast, arterial, and venous.[34] The contrast uptake is measured in Hounsfield units (HU). Parathyroid adenomas have a high HU during the arterial phase (**Fig. 8**) and a lower HU

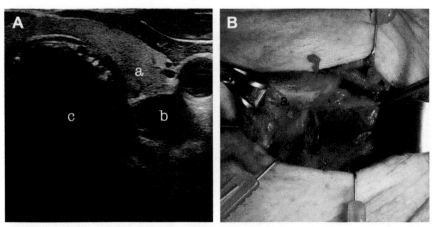

Fig. 7. (*A*) Parathyroid US in axial plane. (*B*) Intraoperative image of the same parathyroid adenoma. a, left thyroid lobe (retracted medially in [*B*]); b, left inferior parathyroid adenoma (retracted laterally in [*B*]); c, trachea; d, RLN. (*Courtesy of* Joseph Sniezek, MD, Swedish Cancer Institute, Seattle, WA; with permission.)

during the venous phase. In comparison, lymph nodes have a very slow uptake and washout, so the HU of lymph nodes are still increasing during the washout phase of a parathyroid adenoma. Because the thyroid gland already contains iodine, it often has a higher HU during the noncontrast phase compared with parathyroids or lymph nodes. Based on these principles, 4DCT is a very helpful second-line imaging modality for some patients: those with a nondiagnostic sestamibi or US; when the sestamibi and US do not correlate with each other; or if the patient will be having repeat or revision surgery. The sensitivity for 4DCT for hyperfunctioning parathyroid tissue is reported to be as high at 87%.[27,28,34]

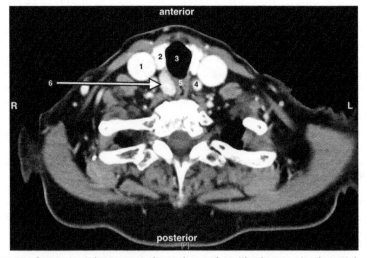

Fig. 8. 4DCT of ectopic right paraesophageal parathyroid adenoma in the axial plane. 1, right internal jugular vein; 2, right thyroid lobe; 3, trachea; 4, left common carotid; 5, esophagus; 6, parathyroid adenoma (*large arrow*).

INTRAOPERATIVE TECHNIQUES

During parathyroidectomy, a few intraoperative resources can aid in confirming adequate excision of the abnormal parathyroid glands: intraoperative PTH assay, radioguidance with sestamibi, and pathologic evaluation of excised tissue.

Intraoperative Parathyroid Hormone Assay

PTH has a half-life of about 4 minutes.[35] In the 1990s, surgeons at the University of Miami published that their use of PTH levels intraoperatively confirmed successful removal of hyperfunctioning parathyroid tissue, resulting in shortened operating time. The so-called Miami Criterion are a greater than 50% decrease in preincision or preexcision PTH levels within 10 minutes of gland removal. This criterion has a sensitivity and overall accuracy of more than 97%.[36] The Miami Criterion has been modified by some surgeons to include a decrease of intraoperative PTH (IOPTH) level into the normal range as well. If the IOPTH level does not decrease by 50%, this implies that multigland or residual disease persists, and indicates that a 4-gland exploration/bilateral neck dissection should be pursued. Rapid or quick PTH assays at equipped institutions take about 15 minutes to process.

Radioguided Surgery

Tc99m injected about 90 minutes before surgery is taken up by the hyperfunctioning parathyroid tissue. An intraoperative gamma probe can be used to locate the abnormal parathyroid. Radioguidance is based on the detection of radiotracer counts that are greater than background counts.[37] Background counts are based on nonparathyroid tissue.[38] Typically the thyroid isthmus is used. Using the probe, counts higher than the background count are sought, guiding the surgeon to the abnormal parathyroid glands. Once identified, an in-vivo to background percentage greater than 150% strongly suggests identification of a parathyroid adenoma. Once removed, the parathyroid tissue is placed on top of the probe tip, away from the patient, and the counts are measured again. If the count is 20% greater than the background, the tissue is confirmed to be the abnormal parathyroid.[37] The use of, and opinions about, radioguided surgery are mixed. Many clinicians think that, because the success of first-time parathyroid surgery with preoperative localization studies and IOPTH is greater than 97%, the use of a gamma probe does not add any benefit. The International Workshop does not advocate this technique, particularly for initial exploration.[35]

Pathologic Evaluation

An additional intraoperative tool is pathologist examination of a frozen section of excised tissue to confirm removal of abnormal parathyroid glands. This tool is typically used in conjunction with IOPTH but not with radioguided surgery. Depending on the experience and efficiency of the pathologist, the frozen section results may return before the designated laboratory draw time for IOPTH (10 minutes), and, if the frozen section examination does not confirm abnormal parathyroid, then the surgery (or exploration) can continue and the IOPTH can be postponed until the parathyroid gland is found.

OBSERVATION WITHOUT SURGERY

It is common to diagnose asymptomatic patients who do not meet the indications for surgery or to diagnose those with indications but who decline intervention. So, what is the natural progression of this disease when surgical intervention does not occur? One of the most cited observational studies on the natural history of PHPT, by Rubin and colleagues[39] at Columbia University, investigated 116 patients with PHPT; 59 who underwent parathyroidectomy and 57 who did not. Both groups were followed for 15 years.

One-hundred percent of the 59 patients who elected for parathyroidectomy had normalization of serum calcium level, PTH level, and urinary calcium excretion postoperatively. BMD also increased and remained above the baseline over the 15-year follow-up. Nine of the 59 patients had symptomatic kidney stones before surgery, with none having recurrent stones after parathyroidectomy.

Out of the 57 who did not have surgery, 25% showed evidence of progression of disease, namely worsening hypercalcemia, hypercalciuria, and BMD reductions, by the tenth year of observation. By 15 years, 37% of patients had progression of disease.

SUMMARY

Over the past 50 years, PHPT has evolved from a disease with significant renal and skeletal manifestations to more often being an asymptomatic, incidentally discovered finding. This evolution has challenged the medical and surgical community to provide more stringent guidelines for determining which patients would benefit from treatment. Surgery is still the only curative treatment of PHPT, but pharmacologic management is available for nonsurgical candidates. The role of vitamin D, the true effects on trabecular bone and fracture risk, the potential for medical intervention, and the manifestations on neurocognition and the cardiovascular system are the foci of future research. It is these unknowns and the unpredictable nature of this condition that make hyperparathyroidism a compelling topic in surgical endocrine disease.

REFERENCES

1. Silverberg SJ, Bilezikian JP. Primary hyperparathyroidism, pathophysiology, surgical indications and preoperative workup. In: Randolph G, editor. Surgery of the thyroid and parathyroid glands. Philadelphia: Saunders/Elsevier; 2013. p. 531–8.
2. Silverberg SJ, Bilezikian JP. Primary hyperparathyroidism. In: Jameson JL, De Groot LJ, editors. Endocrinology: adult and pediatric. Philadelphia: Saunders/Elsevier; 2016. p. 1105–24.
3. Fancy T, Gallagher D III, Hornig JD. Surgical anatomy of the thyroid and parathyroid glands. Otolaryngol Clin North Am 2010;43(2):221–7.
4. Tang AL, Steward DL. Developmental and surgical anatomy of the thyroid compartment. In: Terris DL, Duke WS, editors. Thyroid and parathyroid diseases, medical and surgical management. New York: Thieme; 2016. p. 8–15.
5. Akerström G, Malmaeus J, Bergström R. Surgical anatomy of human parathyroid glands. Surgery 1984;95:14–21.
6. Wang C. The anatomic basis of parathyroid surgery. Ann Surg 1976;183(3):271–5.
7. Thompson NW, Eckhauser FE, Harness JK. Anatomy of primary hyperparathyroidism. Surgery 1982;92(5):814–21.
8. Isales CM, Bollag WB. Physiology of the parathyroid glands. In: Terris DL, Duke WS, editors. Thyroid and parathyroid diseases, medical and surgical management. New York: Thieme; 2016. p. 24–30.
9. Bringhurst FR, Demay MB, Kronenberg HM. Hormones and disorders of mineral metabolism. In: Melmed S, Polonsky KS, Larsen PR, et al, editors. Williams textbook of endocrinology. Philadelphia: Elsevier; 2016. p. 1254–322.

10. Jilka RL, Weinstein RS, Parfitt AM, et al. Quantifying osteoblast and osteocyte apoptosis: challenges and rewards. J Bone Miner Res 2007;22(10):1492–501.
11. Dobnig H, Turner RT. Evidence that intermittent treatment with parathyroid hormone increases bone formation in adult rats by activation of bone lining cells. Endocrinology 1995;136(8):3632–8.
12. Kim SW, Pajevic PD, Selig M, et al. Intermittent parathyroid hormone administration converts quiescent lining cells to activate osteoblasts. J Bone Miner Res 2012;27(10):2075–84.
13. Nishida S, Yamaguchi A, Tanizawa T, et al. Increased bone formation by intermittent parathyroid hormone administration is due to the stimulation of proliferation and differentiation of osteoprogenitor cells in bone marrow. Bone 1994;15: 717–23.
14. Holick MF, Binkley NC, Bischoff-Ferrari HA, et al. Evaluation, treatment, and prevention of vitamin D deficiency: an endocrine society clinical practice guideline. J Clin Endocrinol Metab 2011;96(7):1911–30.
15. Silverberg SJ, Shane E, Dempster DW, et al. The effects of vitamin D insufficiency in patients with primary hyperparathyroidism. Am J Med 1999;107(6):561–7.
16. Kini SR. Lesions of the parathyroid glands. In: Kini SR, editor. Thyroid cytopathology, an atlas and text. Philadelphia: Wolters Kluwer; 2015. p. 484–501.
17. Eastell R, Brandi ML, Costa AG, et al. Diagnosis of asymptomatic primary hyperparathyroidism: proceedings of the Fourth International Workshop. J Clin Endocrinol Metab 2014;99(10):3570–9.
18. Cope O. The story of hyperparathyroidism at the Massachusetts General Hospital. N Engl J Med 1966;274(21):1174–82.
19. Silverberg SJ, Shane E, de la Cruz L, et al. Skeletal disease in primary hyperparathyroidism. J Bone Miner Res 1989;4:283–91.
20. Silverberg SJ, Clarke BL, Peacock M, et al. Current issues in the presentation of asymptomatic primary hyperparathyroidism: proceedings of the fourth international workshop. J Clin Endocrinol Metab 2014;99(10):3580–94.
21. Sorensen MD, Duh QY, Grogan RH, et al. Urinary parameters as predictors of primary hyperparathyroidism in patients with nephrolithiasis. J Urol 2012;187: 516–21.
22. Kidney stone analysis. Lab tests online: empower your health. Understand your tests. A public resource on clinical laboratory testing. Available at: https://labtestsonline.org/understanding/analytes/kidney-stone-analysis/tab/test/. Accessed May 15, 2017.
23. Bilezikian JP, Brandi ML, Eastell R, et al. Guidelines for the management of asymptomatic primary hyperparathyroidism: summary statement from the fourth international workshop. J Clin Endocrinol Metab 2014;99(10):3561–9.
24. Insogna KL, Mitnick ME, Stewart AF. Sensitivity of the parathyroid hormone-1,25-dihydroxyvitamin D axis to variations in calcium intake in patients with primary hyperparathyroidism. N Engl J Med 1985;313(18):1126–30.
25. Udelsman R, Lin Z, Donovan P. The superiority of minimally invasive parathyroidectomy based on 1650 consecutive patients with primary hyperparathyroidism. Ann Surg 2011;253:585–91.
26. Van Udelsman B, Udelsman R. Surgery in primary hyperparathyroidism: extensive personal experience. J Clin Densitom 2013;16:54–5.
27. Redmann AJ, Steward DL. Essentials of parathyroid imaging. Operative Techniques in Otolaryngology 2016;27(3):122–8.
28. Johnson NA, Carty SE, Tublin ME. Parathyroid imaging. Radiol Clin North Am 2011;49(3):489–509.

29. Ruda JM, Hollenbeak CS, Stack BC Jr. A systematic review of the diagnosis and treatment of primary hyperparathyroidism from 1995 to 2003. Otolaryngol Head Neck Surg 2005;132(3):359–72.

30. Mitmaker EJ, Grogan RH, Duh QY. Guide to preoperative parathyroid localization testing. In: Randolph G, editor. Surgery of the thyroid and parathyroid glands. Philadelphia: Saunders/Elsevier; 2013. p. 539–45.

31. Steward DL, Danielson GP, Afman CE, et al. Parathyroid adenoma localization: surgeon-performed ultrasound versus sestamibi. Laryngoscope 2006;116(8): 1380–4.

32. Gurney TA, Orloff LA. Otolaryngologist-head and neck surgeon-performed ultrasonography for parathyroid adenoma localization. Laryngoscope 2008;118(2): 243–6.

33. Untch BR, Adam MA, Scheri RP, et al. Surgeon performed ultrasound is superior to 99Tc-sestamibi scanning to localize parathyroid adenomas in patients with primary hyperparathyroidism: results in 516 patients in over 10 years. J Am Coll Surg 2011;212(4):522–31.

34. Hoang JK, Sung WK, Bahl M, et al. How to perform parathyroid 4D CT: tips and traps for technique and interpretation. Radiology 2014;270(1):15–24.

35. Udelsman R, Åkerström G, Biagini C, et al. The surgical management of asymptomatic primary hyperparathyroidism: proceedings of the fourth international workshop. J Clin Endocrinol Metab 2014;99(10):3595–606.

36. Pasupuleti LV, Lee JA. Intraoperative parathyroid hormone assay. In: Terris DL, Duke WS, editors. Thyroid and parathyroid diseases, medical and surgical management. New York: Thieme; 2016. p. 25–229.

37. Adler JT, Stack BC, Chen H. Radio-guided parathyroid exploration. In: Randolph G, editor. Surgery of the thyroid and parathyroid glands. Philadelphia: Saunders/Elsevier; 2013. p. 613–9.

38. Mariani G, Gulec SA, Rubella D, et al. Preoperative localization and radio-guided parathyroid surgery. J Nucl Med 2003;44(9):1443–58.

39. Rubin MR, Bilezikian JP, McMahon DJ, et al. The natural history of primary hyperparathyroidism with or without parathyroid surgery after 15 years. J Clin Endocrinol Metab 2008;93(9):3462–70.

Moving?

Make sure your subscription moves with you!

To notify us of your new address, find your **Clinics Account Number** (located on your mailing label above your name), and contact customer service at:

Email: journalscustomerservice-usa@elsevier.com

800-654-2452 (subscribers in the U.S. & Canada)
314-447-8871 (subscribers outside of the U.S. & Canada)

Fax number: 314-447-8029

Elsevier Health Sciences Division
Subscription Customer Service
3251 Riverport Lane
Maryland Heights, MO 63043

*To ensure uninterrupted delivery of your subscription, please notify us at least 4 weeks in advance of move.

Printed and bound by CPI Group (UK) Ltd, Croydon, CR0 4YY

03/10/2024

01040397-0017